Handbook of Complementary and Alternative Medicine

Handbook of Complementary and Alternative Medicine

Barbara Wheaton

Larsen & Keller
www.larsen-keller.com

Handbook of Complementary and Alternative Medicine
Barbara Wheaton
ISBN: 978-1-64172-634-4 (Hardback)

Larsen & Keller
Published by Larsen and Keller Education,
5 Penn Plaza,
19th Floor,
New York, NY 10001, USA

Cataloging-in-Publication Data

Handbook of complementary and alternative medicine / Barbara Wheaton.
p. cm.
Includes bibliographical references and index.
ISBN 978-1-64172-634-4
1. Alternative medicine. 2. Medicine. 3. Integrative medicine. I. Wheaton, Barbara.
R733 .H36 2022
615.5--dc23

For more information regarding Larsen and Keller Education and its products, please visit the publisher's website www.larsen-keller.com

Table of Contents

Preface

The medical treatments which are used in place of mainstream therapies are known as alternative medicines. It is also known as integrative medicine, traditional medicine and complementary medicine. There are various popular alternative medicine treatments such as acupuncture, chiropractic medicine, herbal medicine and Ayurveda. Acupuncture is a part of traditional Chinese medicine which makes use of sterile needles to stimulate specific point within the body. Chiropractic medicine studies the body's structure and functions in order to manipulate different parts of the body. This can be done to ease pain, help the body to recover naturally and improve body functions. This book provides significant information of this discipline to help develop a good understanding of alternative medicine and related fields. It is a vital tool for all researching and studying this field. Coherent flow of topics, student-friendly language and extensive use of examples make this book an invaluable source of knowledge.

To facilitate a deeper understanding of the contents of this book a short introduction of every chapter is written below:

Chapter 1- Alternative medicine refers to the set of practices whose healing effects are supposed to be the same as medicine. The effects of such practices are not proven by any scientific method. This is an introductory chapter which will introduce briefly all the significant aspects of alternative medicine.

Chapter 2- Some common alternative practices which are followed across the globe include naturopathy, acupressure, Ayurveda, homeopathy, etc. This chapter discusses in detail the theories and methodologies related to these forms of alternative medicine.

Chapter 3- Mind-body medicine refers to a system of medicine which seeks to understand the effect of emotions and mind on the physical health of an organism. The topics elaborated in this chapter such as meditation and biofeedback therapy will help in gaining a better perspective about mind-body medicine.

Chapter 4- Alternative therapies are gaining popularity across the globe. Some of the common alternative therapies such as aromatherapy, reflexology, chiropractic, reiki, shiatsu, etc. have been carefully analyzed in this chapter.

Chapter 5- Herbal medicines are made from plants which are believed to have therapeutic properties. Some of such herbs include aloe vera, ginger, licorice, panax ginseng, etc. This chapter discusses in detail the theories and methodologies related to herbal medicine.

Chapter 6- Osteopathy is the system of alternative medicine that deals with the treatment of medical disorders by strengthening the musculoskeletal framework. A few aspects that fall under its domain include visceral osteopathy, craniosacral therapy, muscle energy technique, etc. This chapter closely examines these aspects of osteopathy to provide an extensive understanding of the subject.

I would like to share the credit of this book with my editorial team who worked tirelessly on this book. I owe the completion of this book to the never-ending support of my family, who supported me throughout the project.

Barbara Wheaton

1

Introduction to Alternative Medicine

Alternative medicine refers to the set of practices whose healing effects are supposed to be the same as medicine. The effects of such practices are not proven by any scientific method. This is an introductory chapter which will introduce briefly all the significant aspects of alternative medicine.

Alternative Medicine is defined as medicine that encompasses any healing practice "that does not fall within the realm of conventional medicine." Commonly cited examples include naturopathy, chiropractic, herbalism, traditional Chinese medicine, Ayurveda, meditation, yoga, biofeedback, hypnosis, homeopathy, acupuncture, and diet-based therapies, in addition to a range of other practices.

Alternative medicine is defined as any practice that is put forward as having the healing effects of medicine, but is not founded on evidence gathered using the scientific method. Standard care is what medical doctors, doctors of osteopathy, and allied health professionals, such as nurses and physical therapists, practice. The field of complementary and alternative medicine is known as CAM. Complementary medicine can be used together with standard medical care. An example is using acupuncture to help with side effects of cancer treatment.

Complementary and Alternative Medicine (CAM) is a broad domain of resources that encompasses health systems, modalities, and practices and their accompanying theories and beliefs, other than those intrinsic to the dominant health system of a particular society or culture in a given historical period. However bear in mind that what are considered complementary or alternative practices in one country may be considered conventional medical practices in another.

Complementary and alternative therapies are classified into five major groups and some overlap:

- Energy medicine is a domain that deals with putative and verifiable energy fields.
- Biologically based practices use substances found in nature such as herbs, foods, vitamins, and other natural substances.
- Manipulative and body-based practices feature manipulation or movement of body parts, such as is done in chiropractic and osteopathic manipulation.

- Mind-body medicine takes a holistic approach to health that explores the interconnection between the mind, body, and spirit. It works under the premise that the mind can affect "bodily functions and symptoms".

Whole medical systems cut across more than one of the other groups; examples include Traditional Chinese medicine and Ayurveda:

- Aromatherapy is when aroma-rich oils are extracted from specific plants. These oils are mixed with other materials like alcohol, oils, lotions etc to give the desired effects on the body.
- Ayurveda is a system of traditional medicine native to India, and practiced in other parts of the world as a form of alternative medicine. Evolving throughout its history, Ayurveda remains an influential system of medicine in South Asia.
- Biofeedback is a form of alternative medicine that involves measuring a subject's quantifiable bodily functions such as skin temperature, sweat gland activity, blood pressure, heart rate, and muscle tension, conveying the information to the patient in real-time.
- Detoxification is an alternative medicine approach which proponents claim rid the body of "toxins", accumulated harmful substances that are alleged to exert a negative effect on individual health. The idea of a good detox diet is to eat pure and natural foods that will aid the function of the lymph, kidneys, and liver.
- Herbalism is a traditional medicinal or folk medicine practice based on the use of plants and plant extracts. Herbalism is also known as botanical medicine, medical herbalism, herbal medicine, herbology, and phytotherapy.
- Holistic health is a philosophy of medical care that views physical and mental aspects of life as closely interconnected and equally important approaches to treatment. While frequently associated with alternative medicine, it is also increasingly used in mainstream medical practice as part of a broad view of patient care.
- Homeopathy is a form of alternative medicine based upon principles first defined by Samuel Hahnemann in 1796. A central thesis of homeopathy is that an ill person can be treated using a substance that can produce, in a healthy person, symptoms similar to those of the illness.
- Home remedies are a treatment to cure a disease or ailment that employs certain spices, vegetables, or other common items. Home remedies may or may not have medicinal properties that treat or cure the disease or ailment in question, as they are typically passed along.

- Reiki is a spiritual practice developed in 1922 by Mikao Usui. After three weeks of fasting and meditating on Mount Kurama, in Japan, Usui claimed to receive the ability of "healing without energy depletion". A portion of the practice, tenohira or palm healing, is used as a form of complementary and alternative medicine (CAM). Tenohira is a technique whereby practitioners believe they are moving "healing energy" (a form of ki) through the palms.
- Traditional Chinese medicine (also known as TCM) includes a range of traditional medical practices originating in China. It is considered a Complementary or Alternative Medical system in much of the western world while remaining as a form of primary care throughout most of Asia.

Many people utilize mainstream medicine for diagnosis and basic information, while turning to alternatives for what they believe to be health-enhancing measures. Studies indicate that alternative approaches are often used in conjunction with conventional medicine. This is referred to by NCCAM as integrative (or integrated) medicine because it "combines treatments from conventional medicine and CAM for which there is some high-quality evidence of safety and effectiveness.

Alternative medicine has been a source of vigorous debate, even over the definition of alternative medicine.

Dietary supplements, their ingredients, safety, and claims, are a continual source of controversy.

In some cases, political issues, mainstream medicine and alternative medicine all collide, such as the case where synthetic drugs are legal but the herbal sources of the same active chemical are banned.

Alternative medicine practices are as diverse in their foundations as in their methodologies. Practices may incorporate or base themselves on traditional medicine, folk knowledge, spiritual beliefs, or newly conceived approaches to healing.

Types of Alternative Medicine

Many different areas make up the practice of complementary and alternative medicine (CAM). In addition, many parts of one field may overlap with the parts of another field. For example, acupuncture is also used in conventional medicine. In the U.S., CAM is used by about 38% of adults and 12% of children. Examples of CAM include:

- Traditional alternative medicine: This field includes the more mainstream and accepted forms of therapy, such as acupuncture, homeopathy, and Oriental practices. These therapies have been practiced for centuries worldwide. Traditional alternative medicine may include:

- Acupuncture,
- Ayurveda,
- Homeopathy,
- Naturopathy,
- Chinese or Oriental medicine.

- Body: Touch has been used in medicine since the early days of medical care. Healing by touch is based on the idea that illness or injury in one area of the body can affect all parts of the body. If, with manual manipulation, the other parts can be brought back to optimum health, the body can fully focus on healing at the site of injury or illness. Body techniques are often combined with those of the mind. Examples of body therapies include:
    - Chiropractic and osteopathic medicine,
    - Massage,
    - Body movement therapies,
    - Tai chi,
    - Yoga.
- Diet and herbs: Over the centuries, man has gone from a simple diet consisting of meats, fruits, vegetables, and grains, to a diet that often consists of foods rich in fats, oils, and complex carbohydrates. Nutritional excess and deficiency have become problems in today's society, both leading to certain chronic diseases. Many dietary and herbal approaches attempt to balance the body's nutritional well-being. Dietary and herbal approaches may include:
    - Dietary supplements,
    - Herbal medicine,
    - Nutrition/diet.
- External energy. Some people believe external energies from objects or other sources directly affect a person's health. An example of external energy therapy is:
    - Electromagnetic therapy,

  - Reiki,
  - Qigong.
- Mind: Even standard or conventional medicine recognizes the power of the connection between mind and body. Studies have found that people heal better if they have good emotional and mental health. Therapies using the mind may include:
  - Meditation,
  - Biofeedback,
  - Hypnosis.
- Senses: Some people believe the senses, touch, sight, hearing, smell, and taste, can affect overall health. Examples of therapies incorporating the senses include:
  - Art, dance, and music,
  - Visualization and guided imagery.

Complementary and alternative healthcare and medical practices (CAM) isare and medical practices (CAM) is a group of diverse medical and health care systems, practices, and products that are not presently considered to be part of conventional medicine. The list of practices that are considered as CAM changes continually as CAM practices and therapies that are proven safe and effective become accepted as the "mainstream" healthcare practices. Today, CAM practices may be grouped within five major domains: alternative medical systems, mind-body interventions, biologically-based treatments, manipulative and body-based methods and energy therapies.

TCM is a system of healing that dates back to 200 B.C. in written form. China, Korea, Japan, India and Vietnam have all developed their own unique versions of traditional medicine. Alternative medicine is commonly categorized together with complementary medicine under the umbrella term "complementary and alternative medicine". Complementary medicine refers to therapies that complement traditional western (or allopathic) medicine and is used together with conventional medicine, and alternative medicine is used in place of conventional medicine. Alternative medicine refers to therapeutic approaches taken in place of traditional medicine and used to treat or ameliorate disease. Integrative medicine refers to combining complementary treatments with conventional care. The basic philosophy of complementary and alternative medicine include holistic care, which focuses on treating a human being as a whole person.

Examples of complementary and alternative medicine healing systems include Ayurveda, which originated in India more than 5,000 years ago, emphasizes a unique cure per individual circumstances. It incorporates treatments including yoga, meditation, massage, diet and herbs; Homeopathy uses minute doses of a substance that causes symptoms to stimulate the body's self-healing response. Naturopathy focuses on non-invasive treatments to help your body do its own healing. Ancient medicines (complementary and alternative medicine treatments) include Chinese, Asian, Pacific Islander, American Indian and Tibetan practices.

Conventional medicine relies on methods proved to be safe and effective with carefully designed trials and research. But, many complementary and alternative treatments lack solid research on which to base sound decisions. The dangers and possible benefits of many complementary and alternative treatments remain unproved.

While the whole medical systems differ in their philosophical approaches to the prevention and treatment of disease, they share a number of common elements. These systems are based on the belief that one's body has the power to heal itself. Healing often involves marshalling multiple techniques that involve the mind, body and spirit. Treatment is often individualized and dependent on the presenting symptoms.

Basic principles of integrative medicine include a partnership between the patient and the practitioner in the healing process, the appropriate use of conventional and alternative methods to facilitate the body's innate healing response, the consideration of all factors that influence health, wellness and disease, including mind, spirit and community as well as body, a philosophy that neither rejects conventional medicine nor accepts alternative medicine uncritically, recognition that good medicine should be based in good science, inquiry driven and open to new paradigms, the use of natural, less invasive interventions whenever possible, the broader concepts of promotion of health and the prevention of illness as well as the treatment of disease. Studies are underway to determine the safety and usefulness of many CAM practices. As research continues, many of the answers about whether these treatments are safe or effective will become clearer.

The use of alternative medicine appears to be increasing. A 1998 study showed that the use of alternative medicine in the USA had risen from 33.8% in 1990 to 42.1% in 1997. The most common CAM therapies used in the USA in 2002 were prayer (45.2%), herbalism (18.9%), breathing meditation (11.6%), meditation (7.6%), chiropractic medicine (7.5%), yoga (5.1%), body work (5.0%), diet-based therapy (3.5%), progressive relaxation (3.0%), mega-vitamin therapy (2.8%) and visualization (2.1%). In the United Kingdom, limited data seem to support the idea that CAM use in the United Kingdom is high and is increasing.

Increasing numbers of medical colleges have started offering courses in alternative medicine. Accredited Naturopathic colleges and universities are increasing in number and popularity in the USA. They offer the most complete medical training in complimentary medicines that is available today. In Britain, no conventional medical schools offer courses that teach the clinical practice of alternative medicine. However, alternative medicine is taught in several unconventional schools as part of their curriculum. Teaching is based mostly on theory and understanding of alternative medicine, with emphasis on being able to communicate with alternative medicine specialists.

Naturopathy (naturopathic medicine) is a whole medical system that has its roots in Germany. It was developed further in the late 19th and early 20th centuries in the United States, where today it is part of CAM. Naturopathy aims to support the body's ability to heal itself through the use of dietary and lifestyle changes together with CAM therapies such as herbs, massage and joint manipulation. Naturopathy is a whole medical system. It views disease as a manifestation of alterations in the processes by which the body naturally heals itself and emphasizes health restoration rather than disease treatment. Naturopathic physicians employ an array of healing practices, including diet and clinical nutrition, homeopathy, acupuncture, herbal medicine, hydrotherapy, spinal and soft-tissue manipulation, physical therapies involving electric currents, ultrasound and light therapy, therapeutic counseling and pharmacology. Today, naturopathy is practiced in a number of countries, including the United States, Canada, Great Britain, Australia and New Zealand.

The acupuncture is being practiced for relief or the prevention of pain and for various other health conditions. Preclinical studies have documented acupuncture's effects, but they have not been able to fully explain how acupuncture works within the framework of the western system of medicine.

Ayurveda, which literally means "the science of life", is a natural healing system developed in India. It is a comprehensive system of medicine that places equal emphasis on the body, mind and spirit, and strives to restore the innate harmony of the individual. Some of the primary Ayurvedic treatments include diet, exercise, meditation, herbs, massage, exposure to sunlight, and controlled breathing, Ayurvedic medications have the potential to be toxic. Most Ayurvedic medications consist of combinations of herbs and other medicines, so it can be challenging to know which ones are having an effect and why.

Other traditional medical systems have been developed by Native American, Aboriginal, African, Middle-Eastern, Tibetan, Central and South American cultures.

Homeopathy is a system of medical theory and practice. Its founder, German physician Samuel Christian Hahnemann, hypothesized that one can select therapies on the basis of how closely symptoms produced by a remedy match the symptoms of the patient's disease. He called this the "principle of similars". Since homeopathy is administered in minute or potentially non-existent material dosages, there is an a priori skepticism in the scientific community about its efficacy.

Traditional oriental medicine emphasizes the proper balance or disturbances of qi (pronounced chi), or vital energy, in health and disease, respectively. Traditional oriental medicine consists of a group of techniques and methods, including acupuncture, herbal medicine, oriental massage and qi gong.

Naturopathy (naturopathic medicine) is a whole medical system that has its roots in Germany. It was affect bodily function and symptoms. Only a subset of mind-body interventions is considered CAM. Many that have a well-documented theoretical basis, for example, patient education and cognitive-behavioral approaches are now considered “mainstream”. On the other hand, meditation, certain uses of hypnosis, dance, music and art therapy and prayer and mental healing are categorized as complementary and alternative.

Biofeedback is a type of mind-body therapy. Using feedback from a variety of monitoring procedures and equipment, a biofeedback specialist will try to teach you to control certain involuntary body responses, such as: brain activity, blood pressure, muscle tension and heart rate. Biofeedback has been shown to be helpful in treating several medical conditions, including asthma, Raynaud’s disease, irritable bowel syndrome, incontinence, headaches, cardiac arrhythmias, high blood pressure, epilepsy, etc.

The term meditation refers to a variety of techniques or practices intended to focus or control attention. Most of them are rooted in Eastern religious or spiritual traditions. These techniques have been used by many different cultures throughout the world for thousands of years.

People have used prayer and other spiritual practices for their own and others’ health concerns for thousands of years. Scientific investigation of these practices has begun quite recently, however, to better understand whether they work; if so, how; and for what diseases/conditions and populations. Many Americans are using prayer and other spiritual practices. Prayer is the therapy most commonly used among all the CAM therapies.

Manipulative and body-based practices include methods that are based on manipulation and the movement of the body. For example, chiropractors focus on the relationship between structure (primarily the spine) and function, and how that relationship affects the preservation and restoration of health, using manipulative therapy as an integral treatment tool. Massage therapists manipulate the soft tissues of the body to normalize those tissues.

Energy therapies focus either on energy fields originating within the body (biofields) or those from other sources (electromagnetic fields). Biofield therapies are intended to affect the energy fields, whose existence is not yet experimentally proven, that surround and penetrate the human body. Some forms of energy therapy manipulate biofields by applying pressure and/or manipulating the body by placing the hands in, or through, these fields. Examples include Qi gong, Reiki, Prana and Therapeutic Touch. Bioelectromagnetic-based therapies involve the unconventional use of electromagnetic fields, such as pulsed fields, magnetic fields or alternating current or direct current fields, to, for example, treat asthma or cancer, or manage pain and migraine headaches.

Hypnosis is an altered state of consciousness. Hypnotherapy has the potential to help relieve the symptoms of a wide variety of diseases and conditions. It can be used independently or along with other treatments.

Natural and biologically-based practices, interventions and products refer to the use of dietary supplements and include herbal, special dietary, orthomolecular and individual biological therapies. Examples include botanicals, animal-derived extracts, vitamins, minerals, fatty acids, amino acids, proteins and prebiotics, Thousands of studies of various dietary supplements have been performed. However, no single supplement has been proven effective in a compelling way.

In India, which is the home of several alternative systems of medicines, Ayurveda, Siddha, Unani and Homeopathy are licenced by the government, despite the lack of reputable scientific evidence. Naturopathy will also be licensed soon because several universities now offer bachelors degrees in it. Other activities such as Panchakarma and massage therapy related to Ayurveda are also licensed by the government now.

About half the general population in developed countries uses CAM. A survey released in May 2004 by the National Center for Complementary and Alternative Medicine, part of the National Institutes of Health in the United States, found that in 2002, 36% of Americans used some form of alternative therapy in the past 12 months, 50% in a lifetime—a category that included yoga, meditation, herbal treatments and the Atkins diet. The majority of individuals (54.9%) used CAM in conjunction with conventional medicine. Most people use CAM to treat and prevent musculoskeletal conditions or other conditions associated with chronic or recurring pain. Women were more likely than men to use CAM. The largest sex differential is seen in the use of mind-body therapies including prayer specifically for health reasons. If prayer was counted as an alternative therapy, the figure rose to 62.1%. 25% of people who use CAM do so because a medical professional suggested it. A British telephone survey by the BBC of 1,209 adults in 1998 shows that around 20% of adults in Britain had used alternative medicine in the past 12 months.

Advocates of alternative medicine hold that the various alternative treatment methods are effective in treating a wide range of major and minor medical conditions, and contend that recently published research proves the effectiveness of specific alternative treatments.

Evidence-based medicine (EBM) applies the scientific method to medical practice, and aims for the ideal that healthcare professionals should make "conscientious, explicit, and judicious use of current best evidence" in their everyday practice. Although advocates of alternative medicine acknowledge that the placebo effect may play a role in the benefits that some receive from alternative therapies, they point out that this does not diminish their validity. They believe that alternative medicine may provide health benefits through patient empowerment, by offering more choices to the public. Researchers who judge treatments using the scientific method are concerned by this viewpoint, since it fails to address the possible inefficacy of alternative treatments.

As long as alternative treatments are used alongside conventional treatments, the majority of medical doctors find most forms of complementary medicine acceptable. Consistent with previous studies, the CDC recently reported that the majority of individuals in the United States (i.e., 54.9%) used CAM in conjunction with conventional medicine.

The issue of alternative medicine interfering with conventional medical practices is minimized when it is turned to only after conventional treatments have been exhausted. Many patients feel that alternative medicine may help in coping with chronic illnesses for which conventional medicine offers no cure, only management. Classifying treatments need to be based on the objectively verifiable criteria of the scientific method evidence-based medicine, i.e. scientifically proven evidence of efficacy (or lack thereof), and not on the changing curricula of various medical schools or social sphere of usage.

Since many alternative remedies have recently found their way into the medical mainstream, there cannot be two kinds of medicine - conventional and alternative. There is only medicine that has been adequately tested and medicine that has not, medicine that works and medicine that may or may not work. Once a treatment has been tested rigorously, it no longer matters whether it was considered alternative at the outset. If it is found to be reasonably safe and effective, it will be accepted.

It is argued that there is no alternative medicine. There is only scientifically proven, evidence-based medicine supported by solid data or unproven medicine, for which scientific evidence is lacking. Whether a therapeutic practice is "Eastern" or "Western", is unconventional or mainstream, or involves mind-body techniques or molecular genetics is largely irrelevant except for historical purposes and cultural interest. As believers in science and evidence, we must focus on fundamental issues—namely, the patient, the target disease or condition, the proposed or practiced treatment, and the need for convincing data on safety and therapeutic efficacy. The Cochrane Collaboration and Edzard Ernst agree that all treatments, whether "mainstream" or "alternative", ought to be held to standards of the scientific method.

Many forms of alternative medicine are rejected by conventional medicine because the efficacy of the treatments has not been demonstrated through double-blind randomized controlled trials; in contrast, conventional drugs reach the market only after such trials have proved their efficacy. A person may attribute symptomatic relief to an otherwise ineffective therapy due to the placebo effect, the natural recovery from or the cyclical nature of an illness (the regression fallacy), or the possibility that the person never originally had a true illness. CAM proponents point out this may also apply in cases where conventional treatments have been used. To this, CAM critics point out that this does not account for conventional medical success in double blind clinical trials.

People should be free to choose whatever method of healthcare they want, but stipulate that people must be informed as to the safety and efficacy of whatever method they choose. People who choose alternative medicine may think they are choosing a safe, effective medicine, while they may only be getting quack remedies. Grapefruit seed extract is an example of quackery when multiple studies demonstrate its universal antimicrobial effect is due to synthetic antimicrobial contamination.

Those who have had success with one alternative therapy for a minor ailment may be convinced of its efficacy and persuaded to extrapolate that success to some other alternative therapy for a more serious, possibly life-threatening illness. For this reason, critics contend that therapies that rely on the placebo effect to define success are very dangerous. Scientifically unsupported health practices can lead individuals to forgo effective treatments and this can be referred to as "opportunity cost". Individuals who spend large amounts of time and money on ineffective treatments may be left with precious little of either, and may forfeit the opportunity to obtain treatments that could be more helpful. More research must be undertaken to prove the effectiveness of complimentary therapies before they can be incorporated in formal medical practice. Sufficient evidence is required for biological or clinical plausibility in order to justify the investment of time and energy in exploring the merits of alternative medicine. After all, human life is precious and no chances can be taken to comprise the health of any individual.

The Impact of Placebo Effect

In alternative medicine, the main question regarding placebo has been whether a given therapy has more than a placebo effect. Just as mainstream medicine ignores the clinical significance of its own placebo effect, the placebo effect of unconventional medicine is disregarded except for polemics.

Efficacious therapy, in one biomedical definition, is therapy that has positive effects greater than those of an indistinguishable dummy treatment in a randomized, controlled trial (RCT). Such specific efficacy is actually a comparative measure: intervention contrasted with placebo. This relative effectiveness, which is estimated by statistical testing, is taken to indicate "authenticity." The clinical significance, that is, the outcome measured by using the patient's original condition as a baseline, is usually a secondary consideration for determining "legitimate" medical interventions. Any clinical impact due to the placebo, which is deemed to lack "truthfulness," is even less notable and is valued only as a comparison baseline for "genuine" effects. Specific effects are by definition superior to nonspecific effects. The clinical repercussions of the placebo are tolerated as necessary nuisance noise but are otherwise considered inconsequential or treated with contempt.

Given the privileged status of specific effects, it is not surprising that the clinical impact of alternative medicine's placebo effects are routinely ignored. The only serious question has been whether alternative medicine has more than a placebo effect. Discarding all placebo effects in a single trash basket of "untruthfulness," however, diminishes our knowledge of important dimensions of health care. This essay examines the neglected clinical significance of the placebo effect in alternative medicine and raises the possibility that some types of unconventional medicine may produce placebo outcomes that are dramatic and, from the patient's perspective, especially compelling. The term placebo effect is taken to mean not only the narrow effect of an imitation intervention but also the broad amalgam of nonspecific effects present in any patient–practitioner relationship, including attention; communication of concern; intense monitoring; diagnostic procedures; labeling of complaint; and alterations produced in a patient's expectancy, anxiety, and relationship to the illness. The question arises whether alternative medicine can have an "enhanced" placebo effect In some conditions, can any of alternative medicine's particular rituals have a greater impact than the rituals of conventional medicine or than a proven physiologically active treatment? After all, as many of the examples will demonstrate, "two interventions may have different effects on patient outcome even though both are equivalent to placebo in clinical trials". Dismissing a treatment as "just a placebo" may not be enough.

Alternative medicine may be an especially successful placebo-generating health care system. Rather than specific biological consequences, which epidemiologists designate as "fastidious efficacy", alternative medicine may administer an especially large dose of what anthropologists call "performative efficacy". Performative efficacy relies on the power of belief, imagination, symbols, meaning, expectation, persuasion, and self-relationship. We will take components of the placebo drama—patient, practitioner, patient–practitioner interaction, nature of the illness, and treatment and setting— and examines their "placebogenic" potentials in unconventional healing practices. Much of the evidence is derived from conventional research and is speculatively applied to alternative medicine. Also, it should be noted that most of the placebo research discussed does not represent an "artifactual" placebo effect explainable by natural history or regression to the mean. Rather, it usually involves comparative experiments with two different types of placebo or the same placebo delivered under different cognitive or emotional circumstances where two distinct placebo outcomes would not support the idea of placebo effect as only natural history. Obviously, the placebo effect is likely to be at least as heterogeneous in alternative medicine as in conventional medicine, but it is hoped that raising these questions will encourage further discussion and research.

Patient Characteristics

Although the patient is the protagonist in the placebo drama, research has failed to find consistent placebo responders or to identify personality traits or other qualities of persons who frequently react to placebo. However, evidence shows that patient expectations influence outcomes of both placebo and active treatment. Asthmatic patients who believe that an inert substance is a bronchodilator or a bronchoconstrictor respond accordingly. In a small but classic crossover experiment, healthy volunteers received a placebo pill in which a magnet was embedded. In random order, at different times, they were told that they were receiving a relaxant, a stimulant, or a placebo. Subsequent gastric motility was significantly consistent with patients' expectations. Patient expectancies also significantly change or even reverse the actions of many potent pharmaceutical agents.

Adherence to placebo may also be a surrogate marker for a patient's own contribution to the activation of the placebo response. In RCTs, such "placebo adherence effects"—the post hoc differences observed in the placebo arm between those who comply with taking placebo and those who do not—are associated not only with symptom relief but also with concrete end points, including survival. Indeed, differences in adherence are associated with differences in outcomes that exceed the effects of many pharmaceutical agents. Patient preferences for one type of intervention, especially in participative interventions (for example, exercise or diet programs), may contribute significantly to outcomes, including increased placebo responses.

In contrast to conventional medicine, with its measured objectivity, alternative medicine offers a charged constellation of expectations. Alternative medicine's romantic vision is inhabited by benevolent and intentional forces (for example, the innate intelligence of chiropractic or the qi of acupuncture) that are unrestrained by the laws of normative physics. An exaggerated notion of the possible readily elicits patients' magical anticipation. These unconventional concepts do not require absolute belief "in the sense that their truth value is certified by logic or argument" but rather requires moderate openness "in the sense that they are taken into the imagination and lived with, if only for a time".

Alternative medicine emphasizes personal responsibility, which can facilitate adherence. Indeed, the act of switching to another medical system and exhibiting preference by action demonstrates an openness to active participation and adherence and possibly enhances it. Paying out-of-pocket and other signs of commitment, such as following daily lifestyle regimens, undoubtedly marshal adherence effects. The reasons that patients choose alternative medicine may also potentiate a placebo response. Patients with chronic diseases often turn to unconventional healing after long-term negative conditioning with mainstream medicine. In this situation, patients' hope (based on no previous experience with alternative medicine) may provide an opportunity for "deconditioning" from previous unsuccessful medical experiences.

Practitioner Characteristics

The practitioner-healer must expertly play the role of heroic rescuer to facilitate a placebo effect. Numerous RCTs have compared optimistic or enthusiastic physician attitudes toward drug or placebo with neutral or doubtful physician attitudes. Practitioners have had significant impact on such clinical conditions as pain, psychiatric illness, hypertension, obesity, and perimenopause symptoms. Although some studies have shown no effect of physicians' expectations on clinical end points, a systematic review of 85 studies found that although more research is needed, provider-induced "expectancies are a mechanism for placebo effects, which have received support across a range of clinical areas in a variety of studies". A second review, which used more stringent entry criteria, found 25 RCTs that examined the impact of randomly assigning patients with physical illnesses to different levels of expectancy and emotional support. Although researchers found inconsistent effects and determined that further research was needed, they also found that "enhancing patients' expectations through positive information about the treatment or illness, while providing support or reassurance, seemed to significantly influence health outcomes".

Even in blinded RCTs, practitioner certitude seems to influence the magnitude of the placebo effect. In one RCT that simultaneously compared two double-blind RCTs, dental patients in one trial received placebo, narcotic analgesics, or narcotic antagonists and those in the other trial received only a placebo or a narcotic antagonist. Dentists knew the possible interventions in both trials but remained blinded to administration of medication. Pain in placebo recipients was significantly worse in the second trial, in which narcotic drugs were not an option, than in the first trial. An earlier RCT of the effect of physician expectations on hypertension drugs also found that practitioner belief can transform outcomes.

Practitioners of unconventional medicine are less restrained by scientific objectivity than practitioners of conventional medicine. The sensibilities of alternative practitioners are therefore often more optimistic and positive than those of their mainstream counterparts. The characteristics thought to enhance the placebo effect (and any active intervention) seem to be fully operational in the offices of alternative medicine.

Patient Practitioner Interaction

The placebo drama is probably more successful if the patient and practitioner find each other's beliefs and actions mutually credible or at least intriguing. Recipro cal expectations need to be negotiated and joined in the patient–physician duet. Many studies indicate that the patient–practitioner encounter is a potent factor in health outcomes and that for many non–lifethreatening illnesses, clear diagnosis, assurance of recovery, opportunity for dialogue, and physician–patient agreement about the nature of the problem hasten recovery or relief. One study examined 200 patients who presented to general practitioners with symptoms but no abnormal physical signs and in whom no definite diagnosis could be made. Patients were randomly assigned in a 2 × 2 design to treatment or no treatment and to a positive consultation, in which they received "a firm diagnosis and were told confidently that they would be better in a few days," or a negative consultation, in which they were told that their condition was uncertain. Although provision of treatment made no difference, positive interaction produced significantly faster recovery. A similar experiment in 100 patients with acute tonsillitis had analogous results.

Consultation in unconventional medicine is more likely than its mainstream counterpart to produce a precise diagnosis that matches patients' perceptions. In unconventional medicine, patient experience is never devalued or brushed aside as unreliable. Inevitably, since the alternative world is not as constrained by the dichotomy of objectivity and subjectivity, the chiropractor will find the subluxation, the acupuncturist will detect the yin–yang disharmony, and the health food advocate will identify the transgression that makes sense of the patient's life-world. In addition, if a patient is new to alternative medicine, an opportunity for exchange is invariably offered, providing the patient with "theoretical explanations designed to take the mystery out of process and problems". When it is considered that 40% to 60% of patients may never receive a firm diagnosis in conventional medicine, an alternative diagnosis may be a potent form of nonspecific healing that changes the circumstances under which the patient exists, including reducing the "dysphoria of uncertainty".

Besides diagnosis, the healing encounter also establishes therapeutic goals. Paradoxically, while the alternative diagnosis tends to be precise, treatment aims can be diverse. Because of such notions as "holistic medicine" and "body, mind, spirit," alternative medicine can have extremely broad, indeterminate therapeutic targets and therefore, at least from a cultural view, "in some sense cannot fail". Such amorphous goals can provide additional maneuvering room for positive progress, or at least incremental change. If the patient's symptoms do not directly improve, it is likely that something positive will happen and be attributed to the intervention (even if the change pertains only to alternative constructs, such as the homeopathic spiritual force or the acupuncture qi). Taken together, the alternative diagnosis, prognosis, and treatment aims serve "to regulate symptom intensity and distress" and "create enough certainty to diminish the threat of the inchoate while preserving enough ambiguity to allow for fresh improvisation".

The Nature of the Illness

The placebo effect may benefit from the types of illnesses that alternative medicine commonly treats. Data indicate that the overwhelming majority of medical conditions treated by unconventional medicine fall into the following categories: highly subjective symptoms lacking identifiable physiologic correlates, chronic conditions with a fluctuating course often influenced by selective attention, and affective disorders. Not surprisingly, these conditions are precisely those that researchers believe are especially susceptible to inordinately strong placebo responses: back and chronic pain, fatigue, arthritis headache, allergies, hypertension (in some situations), insomnia, asthma, chronic digestive disorders depression, and anxiety. Even researchers who question the existence or significance of a placebo effect—at least in the narrow sense of the outcome produced by a dummy intervention—concede its impact when outcomes are continuous and subjective. Also, persons with self-limiting diseases, such as the common cold and sprains and strains, also frequently use alternative medicine. In these cases, the natural course of the disease undoubtedly creates the appearance of treatment response and enhances the perception of unconventional medicine's effectiveness.

Treatment and Setting

Treatment paraphernalia and setting affect the impact of a placebo performance. For placebo pills, a regimen of four times per day seems more effective than a regimen of twice per day. A "brand-name" therapy that includes either active or inert ingredients may often yield better results than an identical treatment that is not as well known, and devices or elaborate procedures can have greater placebo effects than pills. Active placebos (placebos containing medications, such as atropine, that are ineffective for the condition being studied but produce recognizable drug-related side effects) seem to provide genuine treatment recognition that leads to heightened placebo effects. With good showmanship, a well-designed, totally inert stage prop can offer this kind of "feedback loop" and can produce exaggerated placebo effects.

Two RCTs—one of transcutaneous electrical nerve stimulation and one of "placebo electronic machines"— demonstrated that, with good staging, blank machines can provide feedback sensations. In the first study, all patients reported an electrical sensation after adjustment of the dummy apparatus, which was equipped with visual and sound feedback. In the second trial (which used only dummy machines under two different sets of expectations), a significant number of participants "felt" the nonexistent current, and some even volunteered that the sensation was "just amazing".

Biomedicine and alternative medicine each have a special allure of mystery and exotic power; it would be hard to argue that one backdrop consistently provides a superior placebo effect. However, alternative medicine has the advantage of always having an intervention scenario. Therapeutic passivity is rarely an option, and practitioners can, at a minimum, offer something that is likely to have a placebo effect. In some situations, and at least for continuous subjective outcomes, an intervention presumably has a greater effect than no treatment. Also, to demonstrate "active" intervention, alternative medicine treatments have unique feedback loops that are likely to facilitate, if not heighten, substantial placebo responses. For example, chiropractic adjustment often triggers an audible "pop" so that the patient can hear the subluxation being fixed, acupuncturists propagate a sensation of vital energy coursing through invisible meridians, and psychic healers summon tingling vibrations.

Does Alternative Medicine have Enhanced Placebo Effects

Despite the arguments and speculations already presented, there is scant empirical evidence that any particular type of alternative medicine used for any particular condition has an augmented placebo effect. Even concerning the placebo effect in general, the evidence cited earlier is often methodologically weak and limited by small numbers and short follow-up periods. Some social scientists argue that "for the believer in science, medical care that appears to be scientific would provide a superior placebo; for the believer of whatever other cultural system of meaning and values," alternative medicine may "provide a superior placebo". Perhaps biomedicine's effort to eliminate ritual or placebo interventions itself produces an improved placebo effect.

Two examples from RCTs may help readers concretely envision an enhanced placebo effect. In a fourarm crossover RCT involving 44 patients with chronic cervical osteoarthritis of more than 6 months' duration, acupuncture, sham acupuncture, and diazepam were all equivalent and were superior to a placebo pill. In this study, the outcome of the ritual of acupuncture (real and sham acupuncture were not different) equaled the outcome of an effective drug. In a second RCT, which studied spinal manipulation, 256 patients with nonspecific back and neck disorders were randomly assigned to receive manual therapy (the Dutch equivalent of chiropractic), physical therapy, placebo-device therapy with a "detuned" ultrasonography machine and "detuned" short-wave diathermy that emitted sounds and lights, or treatment from a general practitioner. Six weeks of manual therapy and physical therapy were equally and significantly better than the sham machine, which significantly outperformed the general practitioner. It cannot be determined whether the manual and physical therapies had specific treatment effects or simply yielded better placebo effects than the inanimate gadget. Nonetheless, in this experiment, treatment with a sham machine surpassed treatment from a competent physician for relief of low back pain.

To more rigorously test these possible relative nonspecific effects, my colleagues and I are performing a National Institutes of Health–funded RCT that randomly assigns patients with chronic pain to one of two parallel run-in phases. Before entering two subsequent RCTs, one run-in group receives a conventional-appearing placebo pill and the other receives an alternative medicine sham procedure; the main goal of the run-in phases is to detect differing placebo effects. Any confident assertion about a placebo effect enhanced by alternative medicine would probably require many such experiments.

Some may dismiss these types of investigation as useless. After all, a placebo is just a placebo. Others would argue that such avoidance impoverishes and narrows the understanding of what patients receive from alternative medicine (and, by extension, conventional medicine). Even those who doubt the existence or significance of a "narrow" placebo effect seem open to the possibility of "broad" placebo effects embedded in the psychosocial context of the patient–practitioner relationship.

What is Legitimate Healing?

Besides clinical and scientific value, the question of enhanced placebo effects raises complex ethical questions concerning what is "legitimate" healing. What should determine appropriate healing, a patient's improvement from his or her own baseline (clinical significance) or relative improvement compared with a placebo (fastidious efficacy)? As one philosopher of medicine has asked, are results less important than method? Both performative and fastidious efficacy can be measured. Which measurement represents universal science? Which measurement embodies cultural judgment on what is "correct" healing? Are the concerns of the physician identical to those of the patient? Is denying patients with nonspecific back pain treatment with a sham machine an ethical judgment or a scientific judgment? Should a patient with chronic neck pain who cannot take diazepam because of unacceptable side effects be denied acupuncture that may have an "enhanced placebo effect" because such an effect is "bogus"? Who should decide?

Patients' attitudes toward placebo interventions (especially enhanced interventions) probably differ from physicians' attitudes. This distinction is probably most evident in surgery, another field in which a heightened placebo effect is possible, as illustrated by two RCTs that tested implantation of fetal dopaminergic cells for Parkinson disease. Patients with Parkinson disease seem to have a robust placebo response; the biochemical substrate of this response in relation to the release of dopamine in the striatum has recently been shown on positron emission tomography. At the conclusion of one of the two RCTs, patients were unblinded, and half were told they had received sham surgery that had performed the same as real surgery. In the early reports from this study, both groups experienced significant clinical improvement. (The subsequent full report, which included long-term data, reported a less durable placebo effect.) When patients who had received the sham surgery were told that they could not receive the real but now "discredited" surgery, as they had been promised in the informed consent form, 70% were disappointed or "outraged" because of the dramatic benefits they had already received from sham surgery. They wanted the "real" procedure even if it was equivalent to the sham. Of interest, the second RCT, which also found no difference between active and imitation surgery, demonstrated a stable and significant placebo effect after 18 months. For many patients, performative efficacy may be more critical than fastidious efficacy. Obviously, this illustration is not meant to advocate ritualistic surgery. Rather, it is meant to highlight the complex relationship among clinical, scientific, and ethical judgments.

Alternative Medicine and Children

The distinction between CAM and mainstream medicine has lessened as many practices have undergone rigorous research and have been integrated increasingly into mainstream care. For example, guided imagery and massage have been proven to be effective in the treatment of pain and are now included in many tertiary care settings. Since the American Academy of Pediatrics (AAP) convened the Task Force on Complementary and Alternative Medicine in 2000 and since the creation of the NCCAM, these complexities inherent in the definition of CAM have become more problematic. Given the wide usage and general understanding of the term "CAM," it will be used throughout this report. However, the term "CAM" has been replaced increasingly with "holistic" or "integrative" medicine. Holistic medicine refers to patient-centered care that includes consideration of biological, psychological, spiritual, social, and environmental aspects of health. Integrative medicine is relationship-based care that combines mainstream and complementary therapies for which there is some high-quality scientific evidence of safety and effectiveness to promote health for the whole person in the context of his or her family and community. Integrative medicine also reaffirms the importance of the relationship between the practitioner and the patient, emphasizes wellness and the inherent drive toward healing, and focuses on the whole person, using all appropriate therapies to achieve the patient's goals for health and healing.

The AAP Provisional Section on Complementary, Holistic, and Integrative Medicine, established in 2005, also contributed extensively to this report.

The use of CAM in Western medicine has grown dramatically in recent decades. Many CAM therapies, such as herbal remedies, are mainstream or traditional in many parts of the world. The World Health Organization estimates that most of the world's population regularly uses "traditional medicine" such as traditional Chinese medicine (TCM), Ayurvedic medicine, and Native American healing practices.

In the United States, more than one third of adults have used CAM. The total number of visits to CAM providers increased by 47.3%, from 420 million visits in 1990 to 629 million visits in 1997. The number of visits to CAM providers in 1997 exceeded the total number of visits to primary care physicians in the same year. Estimated expenditures for CAM services for adults increased by 45.2% between 1990 and 1997, with a conservative estimate of $21.2 billion spent in 1997. Of that total, out-of-pocket expenses were estimated to be $12.2 billion. This figure exceeded the 1997 out-of-pocket expenditures for all US hospitalizations. More recent studies have described CAM use among adults as high as 62%, with 41% of adults using 2 or more CAM therapies in a 12-month period.

Children and adolescents also are using CAM therapies increasingly. Weighted estimates of the amount paid for pediatric expenditures on CAM visits and remedies were $127 million and $22 million, respectively. An analysis of the 1996 US Medical Expenditure Panel Survey indicated that only 2% of the pediatric population uses CAM. However, an early study of Canadian children reported 11% use of professionally provided CAM therapies, with chiropractic, homeopathy, naturopathy, and acupuncture accounting for 84% of CAM use. Approximately 20% to 40% of healthy children seen in outpatient pediatric clinics and more than 50% of children with chronic, recurrent, and incurable conditions use CAM, almost always in conjunction with mainstream care. The use of CAM is considerably higher in certain groups of children, including children with special health care needs and homeless adolescents, who have a reported use as high as 70%. Use tends to be most common among patients with asthma, attention-deficit/hyperactivity disorder, autism, cancer, cerebral palsy, cystic fibrosis, inflammatory bowel disease, and juvenile rheumatoid arthritis. Presently, there is little research on the effectiveness of most CAM therapies for many of these conditions. The NCCAM funds various studies, but to date, they have not addressed the pediatric population as a priority focus area for research.

Most pediatric patients who receive complementary therapies also receive conventional care. This fact underscores the importance of pediatricians being aware of the necessity to have an open, respectful relationship and clear communication with families. A 2001 policy statement from the AAP Committee on Children With Disabilities, "Counseling Families Who Choose Complementary and Alternative Medicine for Their Child With Chronic Illness or Disability," recognized that the use of CAM is increasing and provides information and guidance for pediatricians when counseling families about CAM.

Patients' Characteristics and Reasons for using CAM

Children who use CAM are more likely to be seeing their pediatrician for an illness, take medication on a regular basis, and have ongoing medical problems. Approximately half of parents/caregivers of children who used CAM saw a CAM provider for themselves. The majority (66%) of parents/caregivers of CAM users had not informed their child's doctor of the use of CAM for their child. There has been no consistent connection between CAM use and parent income, children's gender, or usual source of care, and there have been mixed findings connecting CAM use and parent education level, family ethnicity, insurance coverage, and child's age.

There are various reasons for the growing use of CAM. Many users of CAM reported use "not so much as a result of being dissatisfied with conventional medicine, but largely because they found these health care alternatives to be more congruent with their own values, beliefs, and philosophical orientations toward health and life." Parents' reasons for seeking care for their children from CAM providers included, in decreasing order of frequency, word of mouth, particular treatment was considered effective, fear of drug adverse effects, dissatisfaction with conventional medicine, and the need for more personal attention. In addition, many cultural groups may use CAM because of cultural values and beliefs.

Despite the public's increasing use of CAM therapies and willingness to pay out-of-pocket for these services, health insurers have had difficulty including them in their plans because of variation in credentialing, difficulties with accounting, and because there are so few Current Procedural Terminology (CPT) codes that cover these services. Although there are CPT codes that cover some CAM techniques, CAM providers may find them difficult to implement because of philosophical differences with a system that singles out disease states or organs from the whole person. Some CAM providers use a separate coding system of more than 4000 codes for CAM procedures and supplies, known as the alternative billing concept or "ABC" codes.

Government Response

The Office of Alternative Medicine was established as part of the NIH by congressional mandate in 1992. In 1998, the Office of Alternative Medicine became the NCCAM. The NCCAM has increased its fiscal-year appropriations from $50 million in 1998 to an estimated $123 million in 2006. Total funding by all institutes and centers of the NIH for research and training on CAM and the training of investigators to study CAM exceeded $225 million in 2006, with additional funding being provided by other agencies and philanthropic foundations. Of the approximately 360 NCCAM-funded research projects in 2006, fewer than 5% were related to pediatrics, including research on the effects of massage for preterm infants, probiotics, omega-3 fatty acids, and food allergies. In 2007 and 2008, the AAP Provisional Section on Complementary, Holistic, and Integrative Medicine urged the NCCAM to consider increasing their priorities and funding for pediatric research, education, and information dissemination (Harry Gewanter, MD, verbal communication).

In 2000, the US President and Congress assembled and mandated the White House Commission on Complementary and Alternative Medicine Policy to make administrative and legislative recommendations to maximize the benefits of CAM for Americans. Comprising 20 physicians and other clinicians, CAM providers, and other experts, the commission was charged with developing a report to address the following:

- Education and training of clinicians;
- Research to increase knowledge regarding CAM;
- Provision of reliable information to clinicians and the public;
- Guidelines for appropriate access to and delivery of CAM.

In March 2002, the commission issued its report, which addressed these charges and examined the relevance of CAM to national efforts to promote health, and created a central coordinating office. The report included 29 recommendations and more than 100 action items for federal agencies, Congress, state government, and other groups.

In 2005, at the request of the NIH and the Agency for Healthcare Research and Quality, the Institute of Medicine released the report Complementary and Alternative Medicine in the United States. The report assessed what is known about Americans' reliance on CAM therapies and assisted the NIH in developing research methods and setting priorities for evaluating such products and therapies.

The US Food and Drug Administration (FDA) also has weighed in on CAM-related issues. The Dietary Supplements Health and Education Act of 1994 (DSHEA) amended previous FDA statutes to encompass dietary supplement–specific provisions, including the definition of a "dietary supplement," product safety, nutritional statements and claims, ingredient and nutritional labeling, good manufacturing procedures, and the classification of "new" dietary ingredients.

Under the DSHEA, a dietary supplement is:

- A product (other than tobacco) intended to supplement the diet that bears or contains 1 or more of the following ingredients: a vitamin, a mineral, an herb or other botanical, or an amino acid;
- Intended for ingestion in pill, capsule, tablet, or liquid form;
- Not used as a conventional food or as the sole item of a meal or diet;
- Labeled as a dietary supplement.

This classification of dietary supplements is specifically separate from food or drug categories and, as such, lies outside the jurisdiction of many of the safety and regulatory rules that cover food and drugs.

According to the DSHEA, manufacturers bear the burden of proof of ingredient safety of dietary supplements. However, unlike pharmaceutical preparations, dietary supplements can be marketed without proven safety or efficacy. A manufacturer does not have to provide the FDA with the evidence on which it relies to substantiate safety or effectiveness before or after it markets its products. For new ingredients, the manufacturer is only required to provide evidence to the FDA that the product is "reasonably expected to be safe."

Manufacturers of supplements are not required to report any data on adverse events to the FDA. The FDA can demonstrate that a supplement is unsafe only after it reaches the market. The FDA must prove that the product is unsafe before it can restrict a product's use or take other legal action. The FDA largely relies on the MedWatch voluntary reporting system to collect safety data on dietary supplements.

The DSHEA also regulates third-party literature regarding dietary supplements. Informational materials may be displayed in commercial retail sites provided they are displayed separately from the product, do not contain false or misleading information, and do not promote a specific brand of supplement. Most important, the DSHEA regulates the labeling of dietary supplements. Under this provision, any claims to prevent, treat, or cure a specific disease are expressly prohibited (unless approved by the FDA). Labels can include statements describing the supplement's effects on the "structure and function" or general "well-being" of the body as long as they are truthful and bear the statement, "This statement has not been evaluated by the Food and Drug Administration. This product is not intended to diagnose, treat, cure, or prevent any disease."

Finally, like food products, dietary supplements are allowed to have suggested dosages on the label and must bear nutritional labeling. The label must include the name and quantity of each dietary ingredient, and if the ingredient is botanical in origin, the label must state the part of the plant from which the ingredient is derived.

Physician Awareness, Attitude and Perception

In 1995, the American Medical Association passed a resolution suggesting that its 300 000 members become better informed regarding the practices and techniques of CAM. Many primary care physicians, including pediatricians, recommend and refer patients for complementary therapies. In the 2001 AAP Periodic Survey 49, "Complementary and Alternative Therapies in Pediatric Practice," pediatricians reported that they recognize patients' frequent use of CAM therapies and expressed a strong desire for additional education on CAM topics. Topics of greatest immediate interest included herbs, dietary supplements, special diets, and exercise. More than one third of the pediatricians reported that they or their families used some type of CAM therapy. Of those reporting CAM use, 70% used massage therapy, 21% received chiropractic care, 13.5% consulted a spiritual or religious healer, and 13% had used acupuncture.

A growing number of pediatric generalists and subspecialists have begun to offer complementary therapies and advice as part of their practice. In addition, there is a growing number of academic pediatric integrative medicine programs and new initiatives to promote systematic sharing, support, and dissemination of information to improve collaborative and comprehensive care. These initiatives include the AAP Provisional Section on Complementary, Holistic, and Integrative Medicine; the International Pediatric Integrative Medicine Network; and the Pediatric Complementary and Alternative Medicine Research and Education Network. However, these initiatives may be insufficient to ensure consistent, quality education across the spectrum of medical education. Standardized curricula or content specifications for physician education on CAM therapies should be considered for medical school, residency, and continuing medical education activities.

Common Cam Therapies

As a means of understanding and integrating different modalities encompassing complementary and mainstream therapies, the Kemper model of holistic care has been widely accepted. This paradigm integrates complementary and mainstream therapies into a coherent construct of treatment options. Another model for understanding CAM therapies has been developed by the NCCAM. This framework focuses on CAM rather than integration of therapies. The most common CAM therapies used by infants, children, and adolescents within the NCCAM framework follow. A complete description of all therapies and scientific evidence regarding each of them is beyond the scope of this report.

Biologically based Practices (Use of Vitamins, Herbs, Other Dietary Supplements, Diets and Foods)

According to the NCCAM, biologically based practices include the use of botanicals, animal-derived extracts, vitamins, minerals, fatty acids, amino acids, proteins, prebiotics and probiotics, whole diets, and functional foods. Of these, multivitamins are the most frequently used CAM products by children, with up to 41% reported usage. Among teenagers who use CAM, nearly 75% use herbs and other dietary supplements. Controlled studies have investigated the use of dietary supplements for various conditions including asthma, upper respiratory infections, diarrhea, depression, anxiety, and attention-deficit/hyperactivity disorder. Several studies are in progress, and the research literature is expanding rapidly. For example, the use of probiotics was considered complementary in the mid-1990s but has become mainstream practice in the 21st century as many gastroenterologists recommend and use them in daily practice for patients with inflammatory bowel disease.

There are a number of excellent review articles on the use of herbal products in pediatric populations as well as data on potentially toxic herbal products and herb-drug interactions. Because of regulations differing from those governing the use of pharmaceuticals, there are concerns about the purity and potency of herbal products and other dietary supplements sold in the United States. Product quality is influenced by many factors, including which portion of the plant is used (ie, root, stem, leaves, flowers), the time of harvest (ie, young versus old plants), the handling of the product, and proper identification of the plant. Furthermore, labeling is often inaccurate. To conduct research, the quality of product must be guaranteed, and to compare clinical trials, the similarity of product must be ensured.

Dietary therapies such as the ketogenic diet in the treatment of seizure disorders have become an accepted practice for some health conditions. However, the popularity of other diets has risen to a new level as the prevalence of obesity and metabolic syndrome has increased and traditional exercise and diet "prescriptions" have failed. The macronutrient content of these popular diets varies widely.

Manipulative and Body-based Practices

As defined by the NCCAM, manipulative and body-based practices include chiropractic and osteopathic manipulation, massage therapy, reflexology, Rolfing, Bowen technique, and Trager approach.

Chiropractic care is one of the most common professionally provided CAM practices. It focuses on the relationship between body structure (primarily that of the spine) and bodily function and how that relationship affects health. With more than 50 000 chiropractors licensed in the United States, the number of children visiting chiropractors is substantial and increasing. Recent studies have confirmed that up to 14% of all chiropractic visits were for pediatric patients and that chiropractors were the most common CAM providers visited by children and adolescents. Few randomized, controlled trials (RCTs) have demonstrated significant clinical benefits of chiropractic practices among pediatric patients; additional studies are needed, and parents need to be cautioned not to rely on chiropractic care as the primary treatment for serious conditions such as cancer. Although anecdotal data suggest that severe complications are possible with chiropractic treatment of infants and children, such adverse effects seem to be rare. Further systematic studies are needed to determine the costs, benefits, and safety of this widely used practice.

Massage is another common manipulative practice that is frequently provided at home by parents and by licensed massage therapists and nurses in clinical settings. Massage is now routine practice in many NICUs to promote growth and development in preterm infants. Massage also has been demonstrated to be beneficial in alleviating symptoms from asthma, insomnia, colic, cystic fibrosis, and juvenile rheumatoid arthritis.

Mind-body Medicine

As defined by the NCCAM, mind-body medicine includes diverse practices such as relaxation, visual imagery, tai chi, qi gong, yoga, meditation, prayer, hypnosis, biofeedback, diaphragmatic breathing, progressive muscle relaxation, and cognitive-behavioral therapies. Many of these practices, particularly prayer, are commonly used among adults. In children, popular techniques include prayer, progressive relaxation exercises, meditation, biofeedback, and hypnosis. Hypnotherapy encourages the child to use his or her imagination to improve health and health behaviors.

Guided imagery, hypnosis, and biofeedback have been shown to be effective adjuncts to medical therapy for such common conditions as chronic, acute, and recurrent pain; anxiety and stress disorders; enuresis; encopresis; sleep disorders; autonomic nervous system dysregulation; habitual disorders; attention and learning disorders; asthma; cancer; and diabetes. These therapies generally have few or no adverse effects.

Spiritual healing includes prayer and is the most prevalent complementary therapy in the United States. Spiritual healing is sometimes included under the rubric of mind-body therapies and sometimes under the rubric of biofield or bioenergetic therapies. Eighty-two percent of Americans believe in the healing power of personal prayer, 73% believe that praying for someone else can help cure their illness, and 77% believe that God sometimes intervenes to cure people who have a serious illness. Prayer is used by up to two thirds of parents for their children.

Studies have suggested that spiritual/religious beliefs and practices may contribute to decreased stress and increased sense of well-being and enhanced immune system functioning. RCTs of the clinical therapeutic effects of prayers in pediatrics are lacking. Some states have pursued legal measures against parents seeking to use prayer or spiritual healing as an alternative to conventional medical therapy for children with serious medical problems such as cancer. However, most families view spiritual healing as a personal practice that is complementary to medical care rather than a replacement for it.

Biofield Therapies

According to the NCCAM, biofield therapies are "intended to affect energy fields that purportedly surround and penetrate the human body." These therapies "manipulate biofields by applying pressure and manipulating the body by placing the hands in, or through, these fields." Biofield techniques include acupuncture, homeopathy, polarity therapy, magnet therapy, Japanese Reiki and Johrei, Chinese qi gong, therapeutic touch, healing touch, and spiritual healing.

Perhaps the best known of the noninvasive biofield therapies is therapeutic touch, which is taught in more than 80 nursing schools and provided in numerous hospitals in the United States. Therapeutic touch is a form of energy medicine that has been developed by nurses on the basis of the premise that healing is promoted when the body's energies are in balance. Nurse-healers are trained to identify and treat energy imbalances to improve the patient's well-being.

Studies on the effectiveness of biofield therapies in pediatric populations have been limited, but the therapies are generally safe.

Acupuncture

Acupuncture has been one component of TCM, which also includes herbal remedies, diet, massage, and lifestyle. Today, acupuncture describes a family of procedures involving stimulation of anatomic points on the body by a variety of techniques. American practices of acupuncture incorporate medical traditions from China, Japan, Korea, and other countries. The acupuncture technique that has been most studied scientifically involves penetrating the skin with thin, solid, metallic needles that are manipulated by hand or by electrical stimulation. Variants of needle therapy include stimulation of acupuncture points by vigorous massage (shiatsu), heat (moxibustion), lasers, magnets, gentle massage or pressure (acupressure), or electrical currents.

Acupuncture is used by an increasing number of pediatric patients. A meta-analysis of the use of acupuncture in the treatment of recurrent headaches suggested potential benefit. Additional applications for acupuncture may include nausea, pain, and allergy.

Whole or Traditional Medical Systems

Whole medical systems involve complete systems of theory and practice that have evolved independently from or parallel to conventional Western medicine. They include homeopathy, naturopathic medicine, TCM, Ayurvedic medicine (India's traditional system of medicine), and healing systems of American Indian/Alaska Native, African, Middle Eastern, Tibetan, and other indigenous populations.

Homeopathy

Developed by Samuel Hahnemann in 1790, homeopathy is based on the theory that "like cures like," meaning that small, highly diluted quantities of medicinal substances are given to cure symptoms, when the same substances given at higher or more concentrated doses would actually cause those symptoms. Unlike classic pharmacology, homeopathy follows the theory that the greater the dilution, the greater the potency of the product. In the United States, an estimated 3000 clinicians, including physicians, nurses, chiropractors, naturopaths, and dentists, use homeopathy in their practices. A range of 2% to 10% of children use homeopathic remedies, most often for respiratory problems, teething, otitis media, and other conditions related to the ears, neck, and throat.

The use of complementary and alternative medical (CAM) therapies is increasing considerably in pediatric and adult populations, particularly among affluent and educated persons. About 20% to 30% of general pediatric patients have used 1 or more CAM therapies; use among adolescents ranges from 50% to 75%. Rates among patients with chronic, recurrent, or incurable conditions, such as cancer, asthma, rheumatoid arthritis, and cystic fibrosis, range from 30% to 70%. Parents of hospitalized children, particularly those in neonatal and pediatric intensive care units, report keen interest in providing CAM to their children during hospitalization, but often have not discussed their interest in or use of CAM with their child's physician.

Pediatricians and medical institutions have struggled to adapt to these rapid shifts in culture and patient demand. Most medical schools in the United States and Canada now offer at least 1 course in holistic, complementary, or alternative medicine—these terms being generally interchangeable—and the number and depth of these courses are increasing rapidly. Physicians, including pediatricians, report a high (over 50%) rate of using CAM therapies themselves, and most physicians provide CAM therapies themselves or refer patients to CAM providers. Are physicians pandering to patient demands? Or are there data to suggest that at least for some conditions and some therapies, integrative medicine offers real benefits?

The terms "holistic medicine" and "integrative medicine" describe approaches to patients and therapies, respectively. Holistic medicine refers to caring for the whole patient—body, mind, emotions, and spirit—in the context of the patient's and family's values, culture, and community; this is simply another way of stating the highest ideals of conventional medicine. Integrative medicine refers to considering a broad range of therapies and selecting those that have the best evidence of safety and effectiveness in the context of holistic care. Integrative medicine takes evidence-based medicine 1 step further by including consideration of all possible therapies, not simply those that have been part of mainstream medical practice.

Treatment Goals

Nearly every study of the epidemiologic characteristics of CAM has underscored the fact that only a few patients and families talk with their physicians about their use of CAM therapies. If physicians want to know what families do and what they value, a systematic approach is necessary in taking a history about patients' goals. We consider therapeutic goals in 5 major categories: (1) curing disease, (2) managing or minimizing symptoms, (3) preventing disease, (4) promoting wellness or resilience and minimizing stress or toxins, and (5) achieving inner peace and harmony.

All of these goals are legitimate. To assess in a meaningful way whether a therapy is useful, both clinicians and patients must explicitly understand the goal or goals of treatment. For example, in treating patients in pediatric oncology, acupuncture may be used, not to cure the cancer (goal 1), but to help manage pain and nausea symptoms (goal 2) or to promote a sense of well-being (goals 4 and 5).

Cam Options

The term CAM encompasses a wide range of disparate therapies that often rely on different philosophies, beliefs, assumptions, and practices. Visits with a homeopathic practitioner typically are lengthy and focus on taking an extensive history, whereas visits with a chiropractor may be brief and focused on a physical examination and adjustment procedures. To understand and remember the range of possible therapies in a clinically useful way, we consider the range of therapeutic options in 4 major domains: biochemical, lifestyle, biomechanical, and bioenergetic. Each domain contains several kinds of therapies. For example, biochemical therapies include medications as well as vitamins, herbs, and other dietary supplements. Biomechanical therapies include massage and chiropractic as well as surgery.

Specific Conditions and Therapies

Few clinicians would argue with the tenet that patientfocused, humane, holistic care is the ideal of medicine. Nor would modern physicians disagree on the importance of considering a range of treatment options and using an evidence basis to select those most likely to be beneficial and least costly or harmful. Questions about the effectiveness of CAM tend to focus on the merits of individual therapies for specific conditions and patients rather than the overarching philosophic orientation to patient care.

For the most part, a great deal more evidence is needed to evaluate claims of safety and effectiveness of natural therapies compared with more synthetic medications and surgical approaches. In practice, most pediatricians do not demand rigorous scientific evidence of safety or efficacy before recommending home remedies such as chicken soup, peppermint tea, or vaporizers for children suffering from mild self-limited conditions such as upper respiratory tract infections. On the other hand, common sense demands that more stringent evidence is required for evaluating the effects of more toxic or costly treatments for life-threatening conditions, particularly if effective treatments are already available. As scientific evidence accumulates, therapies considered as CAM may cross the line into mainstream care; this transition appears to be especially easy if financial support and professional advocacy are involved, for example, marketable products or well-organized practitioners.

Dietary Supplements

Probiotics (for example, yoghurt) have proved effective in reducing the severity and duration of diarrhea in healthy children; many pediatricians have begun recommending increased yoghurt intake for children suffering from diarrhea and as prophylaxis for those children assigned to antibiotic therapy. Health food stores are replete with medicinal products (capsules, tablets, and liquids) containing lactobacilli that claim to "support healthy intestinal function" or "maintain a healthy balance of intestinal flora." The effectiveness and optimal dosing of such products for children remain unknown.

For many other dietary supplements (such as Saint-John's-wort to treat depression and echinacea to treat the common cold), there are no published studies on effectiveness for children. Despite the absence of data on pediatric safety and effectiveness, tremendous efforts are being made to market pediatric herbal products, enticing parents and pressuirng pediatricians. Pediatricians are especially likely to be cautious about the hazards of the long-term use of herbs. Over the past 40 years, increasing data about the cumulative toxicity of a herb that had been widely used for medical, religious, and recreational purposes for centuries—tobacco—support this cautious approach. Recent studies evaluating herb-drug interactions with Saint-John's-wort (leading to notable declines in serum concentrations of digoxin and other medications) also suggest the need for careful review of scientific data before casually reassuring patients about using herbs.

Lifestyle Therapies

Mind-body Medicine

Hypnosis is an effective preventive therapy for pediatric migraines, chemotherapy-associated nausea and pain, and several behavioral conditions. Yet, hypnosis and similar mind-body therapies have not been widely disseminated from behavioral pediatrics to general pediatric practice or specialty areas in which it might be useful in reducing procedure-related anxiety and pain. Currently there are no significant market forces (other than patient demand) promoting the use of mind-body therapies. Teaching such practices demands substantial clinician time, which may be worthwhile over the long term but is poorly reimbursed in some health care systems. Additional research is needed on evaluating the long-term cost-effectiveness of mind-body therapies and developing the most effective strategies for disseminating proven therapies into practice.

Biomechanical Therapies

Massage and Chiropractic

Like hypnosis, massage has proved helpful in treating several pediatric conditions. These include low birth weight, pain, asthma, attention deficit hyperactivity disorder, and depression. Moreover, massage is enjoyable, safe, and sought after by patients. Yet, it is seldom among the therapeutic options considered first by pediatricians. Historically, massage has been tainted by its link with the adult entertainment industry, and it may be viewed as self-indulgent rather than medically indicated. Further-more, as with mind-body therapies, the time required to provide services, personnel costs, and questions about long-term benefits are substantial barriers to the wide-spread use of massage therapies for children.

On the other hand, despite that chiropractic is one of the most common alternative therapies sought by families, there is a remarkable absence of randomized controlled clinical trials suggesting that it is a significantly helpful or cost-effective therapy for any major pediatric disease. Unlike hypnosis and massage therapy, chiropractors have formed a strong professional community that has effectively persuaded the public to pay for their services.

Bioenergetic Therapies

Acupuncture

Research on acupuncture is finally penetrating into pediatric practice. Recent studies suggest that certain children readily accept acupuncture as a possible treatment option and that some acupuncturists specialize in treating children. Whether the benefits noted in adult patients (for example, reducing pain and nausea) are also found in children remains to be seen. Although no unique product is marketed and practitioners have not formed an effective professional guild, acupuncture itself has made intriguing inroads into mainstream medicine; it is now provided as a treatment option in approximately a third of pediatric pain treatment programs at academic medical centers in North America. The vast majority of pediatric patients and their families pay out of pocket for acupuncture services, but third-party payment for acupuncture is gradually gaining ground.

Costs and Benefits

There is a widespread assertion that CAM practices are less expensive than mainstream medicine and that using such therapies will lower overall health care costs. This assertion posits that CAM therapies would replace more expensive mainstream therapies rather than being used in addition to mainstream medicine. This assertion has not undergone rigorous testing. In fact, recent data suggest that including complementary therapies as treatment options increases overall health care costs for adults because

CAM therapies are used as "add-ons" rather than replacements. Similar studies have not been reported for children.

Faith and Healing

Faith, spirituality, beliefs, and religion are words which are often used interchangeably. However, each word has a unique meaning. Faith is the inner search for purpose or meaning in life. It is a strong unquestioning conviction that "there is something more than just me". The concept of faith is a universal one, not necessarily related to God. Even artists who are atheists and want to leave behind a legacy through their art have faith in the "more than just me" that is represented by their art. Spirituality refers to the object of faith (God, nature, the supreme power, art, science, etc.) and all the efforts made to connect with the object of faith, such as prayers, trekking, painting or singing. In other words, spirituality is the compass used by people to guide them towards their faith. Religion is the way of life of a community which shares common beliefs, common spiritual pursuits and a common faith. It is clear from these definitions that faith, spirituality and religion are strongly interrelated.

Many studies have demonstrated linkages between faith, spirituality, religion and health. A few observational studies have linked prayers with a reduction in overall mortality, and in deaths due to cardiovascular complications and cancer. Spiritual pursuits have also been demonstrated to slow down the progression of cancer and hasten recovery from acute illness. There are also some studies which have shown that prayers for patients can speed up their recovery from acute illnesses. Religious practices have also been associated with overall mental well-being. Most of these studies, however, are weak, confounding and riddled with biases. A systematic review of the effect of prayers for distant healing did not support the hypothesis that such prayers have any specific therapeutic effect. Though there is only weak evidence that prayers and faith-based practices have a therapeutic effect, the psychological advantages of such interventions cannot be denied.

Faith healing is a method of treating illnesses through the exercise of faith rather than medical methods. Faith healing is usually practised through prayers to gods and deities. All religions have their own faith healing practices. Several researchers have attempted to establish the effectiveness of faith healing practices. Two randomised controlled trials in the USA, which investigated intercessory prayers and their effect on the recovery of patients admitted in the coronary care unit, revealed that the group who were randomised to the prayer had significantly better scores on a composite index of course of illness during hospital stay. Both these studies were limited by the fact that a thorough adjustment for confounders was not done and blinding was not possible. The outcomes that showed a significant difference between the two groups were subjective parameters. Though these facts weaken the argument for the strength of the effects of prayer, these studies show that there is a possible association that needs to be explored further. Several explanations have been proposed for the effectiveness of faith healing. These include psychological benefits, a better response to stress, healthier coping mechanisms and the activation of the immune system. Psychoneuroimmunology and the placebo effect have also been put forward as explanations for this association. However, one of the important reasons why modern medical practitioners hesitate to discuss faith healing with patients is the paradigmatic difference in the approach of modern medicine, which is focused on cure, as against religious and spiritual practices, which are focused on healing. It is important to understand the differences between cure and healing in the context of medical treatment.

Healing versus Cure – The Semantic Dichotomy

Over the years, the outcome of medical endeavours has gradually come to be viewed as "cure" rather than "healing". In historical times, medicine was considered a "healing" profession. With the advances in science and developments in medical technology, the biomedical scientist–physician has become a curer rather than a healer. The biomedical model lends itself to an objective examination of the organs, systems and their functions, attributes diseases to the observations made and attempts cures that are specific to diseases. This approach tends to distance itself from the holistic psychological, emotional and spiritual disturbances associated with diseases.

As for healing, the anthropological literature considers the healing process as a response to illness and classifies it as scientific and faith-based. It also explores the various faith-based healing processes in the western and eastern cultural contexts. The psychology literature looks at healing as "a process in the service of the evolution of the whole personality towards ever greater and more complex wholeness". Nursing literature defines healing as "the process of bringing together aspects of one's self – body–mind–spirit – at deeper levels of inner knowing, leading toward integration and balance, with each aspect having equal importance and value". Healing is a process of transcending suffering in the physical, psychological and spiritual planes. Thus, the narrow biomedical concept of cure should be clearly distinguished from the more holistic concept of healing, which encompasses the physical, mental, social and spiritual.

There is a strong division today between the physician's role as a "curer" and the nurse's role as the "carer". These roles, however, are slowly merging and physicians are increasingly required to take on holistic caring roles. In this context, a more open dialogue on spiritual and faith-based healing becomes essential. Apart from a focus on cure, the biomedical model of health places the physician at the centre of the treatment process. This approach has led to a systematic distancing of patients from doctors, as well as to rising healthcare costs because the physicians who are now at the centre of the treatment process place more emphasis on the disease and its cure rather than on patients and healing them. In an attempt to "cure" patients, they order expensive investigations and treatments, which lead to rising costs of healthcare without paying attention to "healing". An emerging concept that is radically changing this approach is patient-centred care.

Patient-centred Care – Focusing on the Patient

The global discourse on patient-centred care has picked up over recent years. Such care is seen as the ideal, cost-effective and meaningful way of delivering clinical services. Patientcentred care is defined as care which is respectful of and responsive to the individual patient's preferences, needs and values, and which ensures that the patient's values guide all clinical decisions. The fundamental tenet of such care is determining what matters most to a patient. When the patient is placed at the centre of care, there is an increase in the patient's level of satisfaction, an improvement in clinical outcomes, and a reduction in unnecessary diagnostic tests, hospitalisations and treatments which, in turn, brings down the overall cost of healthcare. The process of healing is more important than cure itself because it encompasses care, concern, the involvement of the patient, shared decisionmaking, and psychological, spiritual and emotional support, all of which the patient needs, appreciates and absorbs to heal. With the emerging evidence of a relationship between faith, spirituality and health, evidence of the effectiveness of faith healing practices, consideration of the holistic concept of healing (psycho-socio-spiritual), and moves to place the patient's preferences and requests at the centre of the care process, active engagement with requests for faith healing becomes essential. However, modern medical practitioners do not regularly discuss faith, spiritual pursuits, religious beliefs or practices with their patients. There are several reasons for this.

Factors Influencing Physicians' Approach to their Patients' Faith and Faith Healing Requests

The most important reason why physicians steer clear of discussing faith healing is their lack of knowledge of emerging research and evidence in this area. Approaches to alternative forms of healing do not form a part of the medical curriculum at any level. This creates a general disinterest in, and sometimes disbelief and disrespect for, the alternative forms of healing. Barring a few faith-based medical schools in India, religion is systematically dissociated from medical practice. Medical students are brainwashed into believing that medicine is purely a matter of science and that faith, spirituality and religion have no value in medical practice. These physicians feel uneasy addressing their patients' requests for faith healing. Often, they end up analysing the biomedical benefits of such practices and making ill-informed judgments based on the analysis. For instance, from his biomedical perspective, the uninformed physician looks upon the practice of sprinkling holy water and holy ash on a schizophrenia patient as a faith healing practice, concludes that these have no effect on the dopamine levels in the brain of the patient and hence, are unlikely to produce an effect on the patient. This creates disinterest in and sometimes, disrespect for the faith healing practices. Yet another important reason for failing to engage with those who make requests for faith healing is a perception that such discussions are time-consuming and will waste valuable time during the clinical encounter. The physician's assessment of the severity of a patient's condition will compound this perception of lack of time. Another major reason why physicians distance themselves from faith healing requests is that they have strictly compartmentalised their work, in that they often feel that faith, spirituality and religion are beyond the scope of clinical work and that they are not required to do that work. All these factors may be modified to produce a more balanced approach to requests for faith healing. Medical students can be trained to have an open, albeit critical, approach to alternative forms of healing by increasing their knowledge and exposure to these systems. Educating doctors from the start of their training to be socially, culturally and spiritually competent physicians should be given priority in medical education reforms.

Making an Ethical Choice

However well trained and spiritually competent a physician may be, each request for faith healing comes with a unique set of ethical issues which the physician must consider before making the decision. Is faith healing the only option available to the patient at a cost that he/she can afford? Is the patient being pushed to resort to faith healing because of financial constraints, issues related to access to healthcare, social pressures or caste barriers? Is the request for faith healing a well-informed personal choice based on faith, spiritual practices, beliefs and values? It is important to answer these questions as they address the issue of healthcare inequities versus a well-informed autonomous choice. Trust in faith healers can often be a double-edged sword as it makes the individual who trusts vulnerable to exploitation. Is the faith healer exploiting the patient? This is another very important ethical question that arises while addressing requests for faith healing. Performing a risk–benefit analysis for faith healing practices may not always be possible. A spiritually and culturally sensitive risk–benefit analysis should be attempted. It is important to note that in the context of healing, faithbased practices are not value-neutral and their relative merits and demerits are contextual. The outright rejection or unquestioning acceptance of faith healing requests can communicate a lack of interest and involvement in the patient's well-being. Active inquiry into the patient's faith, spiritual practices and religious beliefs will help set the stage for a discussion on the request for faith healing. The clinical decision on faith healing should be a shared one, one in which the patient's preferences and physician's concerns are discussed openly. A respectful and interested approach to requests for faith healing may not produce miraculous cures, but will surely increase the patient's faith in the process of healing.

The Role of Spirituality in Health Care

The technological advances of the past century tended to change the focus of medicine from a caring, service oriented model to a technological, cure-oriented model. Technology has led to phenomenal advances in medicine and has given us the ability to prolong life. However, in the past few decades physicians have attempted to balance their care by reclaiming medicine's more spiritual roots, recognizing that until modern times spirituality was often linked with health care. Spiritual or compassionate care involves serving the whole person—the physical, emotional, social, and spiritual. Such service is inherently a spiritual activity. Rachel Naomi Remen, MD, who has developed Commonweal retreats for people with cancer, described it well:

> "Helping, fixing, and serving represent three different ways of seeing life. When you help, you see life as weak. When you fix, you see life as broken. When you serve, you see life as whole. Fixing and helping may be the work of the ego, and service the work of the soul".

Serving patients may involve spending time with them, holding their hands, and talking about what is important to them. Patients value these experiences with their physicians. In this topic, I discuss elements of compassionate care, review some research on the role of spirituality in health care, highlight advantages of understanding patients' spirituality, explain ways to practice spiritual care, and summarize some national efforts to incorporate spirituality into medicine.

Compassionate Care: Helping Patients Find Meaning in their Suffering and Addressing their Spirituality

The word compassion means "to suffer with." Compassionate care calls physicians to walk with people in the midst of their pain, to be partners with patients rather than experts dictating information to them.

Victor Frankl, a psychiatrist who wrote of his experiences in a Nazi concentration camp, wrote: "Man is not destroyed by suffering; he is destroyed by suffering without meaning". One of the challenges physicians face is to help people find meaning and acceptance in the midst of suffering and chronic illness. Medical ethicists have reminded us that religion and spirituality form the basis of meaning and purpose for many people. At the same time, while patients struggle with the physical aspects of their disease, they have other pain as well: pain related to mental and spiritual suffering, to an inability to engage the deepest questions of life. Patients may be asking questions such as the following: Why is this happening to me now? What will happen to me after I die? Will my family survive my loss? Will I be missed? Will I be remembered? Is there a God? If so, will he be there for me? Will I have time to finish my life's work? One physician who worked in the pediatric intensive care unit told me about his panic when his patients' parents posed such questions. It is difficult to know what to say; there are no real answers. Nevertheless, people long for their physicians as well as their families and friends to sit with them and support them in their struggle. True healing requires answers to these questions. Cure is not possible for many illnesses, but I firmly believe that there is always room for healing. Healing can be experienced as acceptance of illness and peace with one's life. This healing, I believe, is at its core spiritual.

Two examples illustrate ways to deal with questions related to meaning in life. Many studies have shown that people desire to be remembered. Some wish to fulfill this desire through their family, and others through their life's accomplishments or impact. One of my patients has had ovarian cancer for 7½ years. Recently, the cancer metastasized and is no longer as responsive to chemotherapy. She has been involved in lecturing to a class of my medical students for a 2-week period each semester, talking about medical care from a patient's perspective. Now that she is facing the end of her life, she is determined to continue those lectures; she finds purpose in the significant impact they have had on future physicians. Her treatment team was able to work around certain therapeutic protocols to enable her to achieve her dreams and goals. Another patient was dying of breast and ovarian cancer in her early 30s, and she was depressed. Antidepressants weren't helping. Through talking with her, I understood the cause of her suffering: a fear that her 2-year-old daughter would not remember her. I suggested that she keep a journal to leave to her daughter; the hospice nurses videotaped her messages to her children. These activities helped resolve her depression.

Erik Erikson has written about certain developmental tasks that he suggests children, adolescents, and adults need to accomplish as part of the normal developmental and maturing process. Spirituality has been recognized by many authors as an integral developmental task for those who are dying. Unfortunately, people who are dying are often ignored. DNR—do not resuscitate—is often interpreted as "do not round." As these patients deal with issues of transcendence, they need someone to be present with them and support them in this process. We need to advocate for systems of care in which that can happen.

Attending the dying patient is an important experience for physicians as well. In an article entitled "When mortality calls, don't hang up," Sally Leighton wrote: "The physician will do better to be close by to tune in carefully on what may be transpiring spiritually, both in order to comfort the dying and to broaden his or her own understanding of life at its ending". One Baylor nurse I spoke with said that her patients give back 400% more than she gives them. I have to echo that sentiment. Being in the presence of people who are struggling and are able to transcend suffering and pain and see life in a different way is inspiring for me, and I'm grateful for those experiences.

Research on the Role of Spirituality in Health Care

The effect of spirituality on health is an area of active research right now. Besides being studied by physicians, it is studied by psychologists and other professionals. The studies tend to fall into 3 major areas: mortality, coping, and recovery.

Mortality

Some observational studies suggest that people who have regular spiritual practices tend to live longer. Another study points to a possible mechanism: interleukin (IL)-6. Increased levels of IL-6 are associated with an increased incidence of disease. A research study involving 1700 older adults showed that those who attended church were half as likely to have elevated levels of IL-6. The authors hypothesized that religious commitment may improve stress control by offering better coping mechanisms, richer social support, and the strength of personal values and worldview.

Coping

Patients who are spiritual may utilize their beliefs in coping with illness, pain, and life stresses. Some studies indicate that those who are spiritual tend to have a more positive outlook and a better quality of life. For example, patients with advanced cancer who found comfort from their religious and spiritual beliefs were more satisfied with their lives, were happier, and had less pain. Spirituality is an essential part of the "existential domain" measured in quality-of-life scores. Positive reports on those measures—a meaningful personal existence, fulfillment of life goals, and a feeling that life to that point had been worthwhile— correlated with a good quality of life for patients with advanced disease.

Some studies have also looked at the role of spirituality regarding pain. One study showed that spiritual well-being was related to the ability to enjoy life even in the midst of symptoms, including pain. This suggests that spirituality may be an important clinical target. Results of a pain questionnaire distributed by the American Pain Society to hospitalized patients showed that personal prayer was the most commonly used non-drug method of controlling pain: 76% of the patients made use of it. In this study, prayer as a method of pain management was used more frequently than intravenous pain medication (66%), pain injections (62%), relaxation (33%), touch (19%), and massage (9%). Pain medication is very important and should be used, but it is worthwhile to consider other ways to deal with pain as well.

Spiritual beliefs can help patients cope with disease and face death. When asked what helped them cope with their gynecologic cancer, 93% of 108 women cited spiritual beliefs. In addition, 75% of these patients stated that religion had a significant place in their lives, and 49% said they had become more spiritual after their diagnosis. Among 90 HIV-positive patients, those who were spiritually active had less fear of death and less guilt. A random Gallup poll asked people what concerns they would have if they were dying. Their top issues were finding companionship and spiritual comfort—chosen over such things as advance directives, economic/financial concerns, and social concerns. Those who were surveyed cited several spiritual reassurances that would give them comfort. The most common spiritual reassurances cited were beliefs that they would be in the loving presence of God or a higher power, that death was not the end but a passage, and that they would live on through their children and descendants.

Bereavement is one of life's greatest stresses. A study of 145 parents whose children had died of cancer found that 80% received comfort from their religious beliefs 1 year after their child's death. Those parents had better physiologic and emotional adjustment. In addition, 40% of those parents reported a strengthening of their own religious commitment over the course of the year prior to their child's death.

These findings are not surprising. We hear them repeated in focus groups, in patients' writings and stories: When people are challenged by something like a serious illness or loss, they frequently turn to spiritual values to help them cope with or understand their illness or loss.

Recovery

Spiritual commitment tends to enhance recovery from illness and surgery. For example, a study of heart transplant patients showed that those who participated in religious activities and said their beliefs were important complied better with follow-up treatment, had improved physical functioning at the 12-month follow-up visit, had higher levels of self-esteem, and had less anxiety and fewer health worries. In general, people who don't worry as much tend to have better health outcomes. Maybe spirituality enables people to worry less, to let go and live in the present moment.

Related to spirituality is the power of hope and positive thinking. In 1955, Beecher showed that between 16% and 60% of patients—an average of 35%—benefited from receiving a placebo for pain, cough, drug-induced mood change, headaches, seasickness, or the common cold when told that the placebo was a drug for their condition. Now placebos are used only in clinical trials, and even there, generally about 35% of people respond to them. Study of the "placebo effect" has led to conclusions that our beliefs are powerful and can influence our health outcomes. Herbert Benson, MD, a cardiologist at Harvard School of Medicine, has renamed the placebo effect "remembered wellness". You see this as an ability to tap into one's inner resources to heal. Benson, yourself, and others see the physician-patient relationship as having placebo effect as well—i.e., the relationship itself is an important part of the therapeutic process. Benson suggests that there are 3 components that contribute to the placebo effect of the patient-physician relationship: positive beliefs and expectations on the part of the patients, positive beliefs and expectations on the part of the physician or health care professional, and a good relationship between the 2 parties.

Specific spiritual practices have been shown to improve health outcomes. In the 1960s, Benson began research on the effect of spiritual practices on health. Some people who practiced transcendental meditation approached him in the 1960s and asked him to determine if meditation had beneficial health effects. He found that 10 to 20 minutes of meditation twice a day leads to decreased metabolism, decreased heart rate, decreased respiratory rate, and slower brain waves. Further, the practice was beneficial for the treatment of chronic pain, insomnia, anxiety, hostility, depression, premenstrual syndrome, and infertility and was a useful adjunct to treatment for patients with cancer or

HIV. He called this "the relaxation response." Benson concluded: "To the extent that any disease is caused or made worse by stress, to that extent evoking the relaxation response is effective therapy".

Challenges to Alternative Medicine

Precisely because practices have some traits that make them "alternative" that they have not been studied, are not used in hospitals or taught in medical schools, and are not reimbursed by healthcare insurance companies, and not vice versa, as is implied in the current definitions of AM. As asserted above, the requirements of science are not the only reason why AM is deemed "alternative." A number of other factors have played a role, either to keep these practices out of mainstream healthcare or, on the contrary, to draw attention to them, and encourage considering them as potential therapeutic options. Below, we discuss briefly political, economic, scientific and social factors influencing understanding and integration of AM.

Political and Regulatory Factors

The interaction of politics and healthcare is extensive, complex, and inevitable because healthcare is such a fundamental aspect of national economies, and because individual and population health status must be addressed.

For example, political interventions, as suggested above, have played a significant role in AM's recent development in the US. In October 1991, the US Congress directed the NIH to create an Office of Unconventional Medical Practices. This was met with a less-than-enthusiastic response from this government agency, but simultaneously, with high public expectations. The public and congress have consistently put pressure on the Office of Alternative Medicine (now the NCCAM) to fulfill its mandate, while the NIH has been reluctant to progress too fast in a field that it does not consider "scientific."

In most countries, politics are similarly involved at some level of the development of alternative or traditional medicine. For example, in the People's Republic of China, the Chinese Administration of Traditional Chinese Medicine is under the authority of the Chinese Ministry of Health. The Chinese government has been active in guiding the modernization of technological and scientific approaches to TCM. This has brought much better standards to the quality control of TCM botanical medicine preparations so that they can enter the international market and compete effectively with other botanical medicine preparations, in particular those from Europe.

On the other hand, in Singapore, where scientific biomedicine is the standard of care, the government has only recently expressed interest in acupuncture, and only in the context of scientifically documenting that therapy's effectiveness prior to allowing its official use.

This process also drew attention to the fact that TCM was being used by approximately half the population and practiced by a significant number of practitioners, while there were no regulations, neither for practitioner qualification nor to ensure quality of the products.

Regulatory issues are a subset of political issues, as regulations are a product of government agencies. In the US, the Food and Drug Administration (FDA) oversees products and devices used in the practice of medicine. For complex political and legal reasons too long to detail here, botanical medicines and dietary supplements have become essentially unregulated. They need not meet qualitycontrol standards, and significant information need not be provided on the packaging of these products, which may put the public at risk.

It is difficult to apply to alternative medical products the same regulations as those applied to biomedical products and devices, in particular to those used in traditional practices from other cultures. The lack of appropriate US regulations for alternative medical products reflects this difficulty. There are several reasons for this. For example, many traditional practices follow different diagnostic classifications compare to biomedicine. In addition, the complex substances (e.g., botanical, animal products) they use cannot easily meet the criteria established for essentially pure drugs, or even for conventional biologics. However, recently, the FDA has begun addressing the issues posed by AM product evaluation. In particular, FDA representatives actively participated in the organization of two conferences that addressed the special considerations of acupuncture and of botanical medicines.

Economic Factors

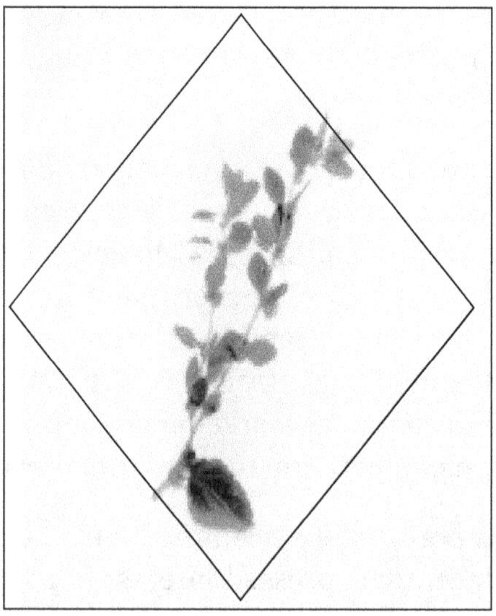

In most countries, the economic potential of growing AM markets has meant that much business and research interest in AM to date has been focused on specific techniques and products that can be marketed. On the other hand, the "healthcare industry," or even academia, have rarely paid attention to conceptual and philosophical principles on which the use of those products and techniques are based. This trend is even reflected in government-sponsored research.

In countries like Peru, the government's interest in traditional medicine began mostly in the context of providing affordable healthcare for indigenous populations, for example, in the Amazon basin where most people are too poor to afford costly Western medicine, and too remote to have access to it. However, in these countries also, the new interest in specific products (e.g., "cat's claw," "camu-camu" and "sangre de grado") by the herbal medicine industry is beginning to create incentives other than those of affordable and accessible healthcare for the indigenous populations. These new economic incentives may be counter-productive: they may endanger both the survival of the plant species and, consequently, the health of the indigenous populations, because they encourage an economically needy population to over-harvest (perhaps to extinction) plants on which they may need to rely on for their own health.

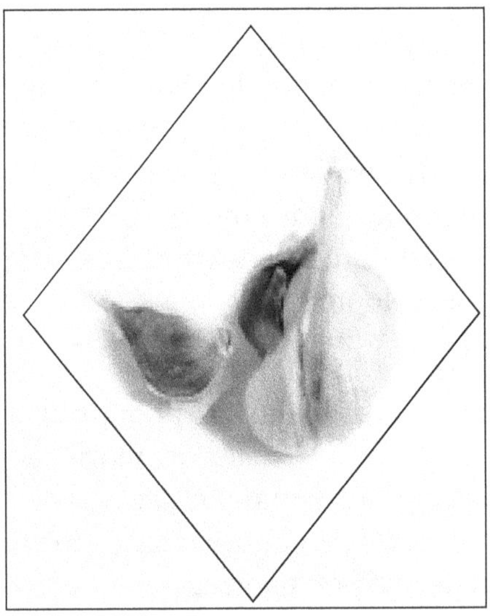

In China, the government has launched a program implementing schedules for the development of new TCM "products." Government and academic representatives have visited the US to indicate their eagerness to collaborate and to follow proper methodology (e.g. double blind randomized clinical trials (RCT)). Recently, at such a meeting, it was recognized that traditional Chinese "medicine" should be distinguished from TCM "products."

In the US, the "healthcare industry", as the major players define it, is one of the most lucrative American enterprises. As documented in several recent reports, a large proportion of the American population use alternative medicine and therefore constitutes a considerable potential market in the US. Consequently, alternative practices and products that had been shunned by the traditional healthcare industry are becoming an increasingly promoted feature of American healthcare packages, from healthcare maintenance organizations to hospitals, including academically affiliated ones. In 1999, two major "first of their kind" conferences were held, cosponsored by academic medical center AM units and private "integrative medicine" entities, to educate not so much professionals and researchers, but mostly hospital, HMO, and insurance executives and administrators about how to integrate AM practices and products into their institutions and services. It is laudable that a wider community will become informed, but will the adoption of "complementary care," as it is sometimes called, truly lead to changes in the practice of medicine? The fact that the NCCAM is beginning to sponsor a few large clinical trials (e.g., St. John's wort for the treatment of depression, glucosamine for the treatment of arthritis), also stresses an emphasis on products and disease rather than on conceptual and philosophical approaches to maintaining health.

The large and rapidly growing market for AM has created the potential for substantial financial gain, but a quick "pay off" may yield research of poor quality, and perpetuate research only aimed at narrowly evaluating products' effectiveness. While it is important to conduct such research, this may also lead to botanical medicine being used in the same manner as conventional drugs, as "magic bullets" for the treatment of specific medical conditions. However, because whole plants themselves are difficult to patent, there is strong financial incentive to attempt to identify active ingredients only, or at least standardized and relatively purified ones, whereas a well-rounded regimen of botanical medicine may involve whole plants and/or combinations thereof. Study of other benefits to be derived from traditional systems of health must go hand-in-hand with botanical and other product development.

Finally, we have additional reasons to want to explore options other than "magic bullet" drugs. Frequent reports now sound the alarm about our escalating, critical problem with drug interactions. In the West in particular, more people take more "magic bullets" than ever before, in part because many older people have chronic ills requiring many medications. We must understand other routes to creation and maintenance of health with diminished reliance on polypharmacy.

Scientific Factors

Science is not a field of study but a method of observation that must be tailored to the object (or phenomenon) being studied. In this context, any phenomenon may be worthy of study, provided there is a phenomenon to study. Many factors can determine whether an area is worthy of study — for example, potential scientific significance of positive or even negative findings; strength of evidence to date; theoretical or methodological "hot topics"; technological impediments or breakthroughs; societal or scientific needs or biases. Scientists largely investigate within constraints of available funding, but it is also the responsibility of the scientific community to be mindful of the above issues. Scientists must also tailor the means of observation (the scientific method) to the subject, rather than a standard method of observation and then try to fit the object of study within the method that may deform (sometimes beyond recognition) the subject being studied.

In general there are many methodological approaches to the study of alternative or traditional medicine, and there is no restriction as to which one can be used. However, one must be very careful about the interpretation and extrapolation of results. For example, a number of double blind studies have been conducted on acupuncture for nausea, using a single point, "Pericardium 6" (P6). This series of generally well-designed studies has indicated that the stimulation by a needle of a traditional acupoint (P6) can affect a centrally controlled symptom (nausea), and that this effect is specific since needling of another point does not have any effect. Thus, these results give credence to the basic premise of acupuncture. However, in our opinion, this series of studies does not evaluate the effectiveness of acupuncture, as, in most instances, acupuncturists would not needle a single point, regardless of other accompanying signs and symptoms.

While science claims to be dispassionate, many scientists have become polarized around the issue of alternative medicine. For decades, Western academia has excluded research and practice in areas identified with AM, and has shunned those who dared defy the status quo. This opposition has contributed substantially to the paucity of data in this area. For example, in the US, established academics have been discredited and have had difficulties when attempting to do AM research, and at times, explicit threats were made by mainstream medicine to individuals and institutions that would associate with alternative practitioners, or who would do research in areas identified as alternative. Consequently, most AM research is conducted outside of academia by individuals with limited research training and resources, and their investigations are often methodologically inadequate. Conversely, those AM studies deemed methodologically sound may lack comparability and replicability. For example, lack of funding and differences among individual investigators' resources and personal research interests have limited replication of hundreds of studies in homeopathy and acupuncture.

In summary, we believe that the scientific method can and must be applied to the study of traditional medicine. However, we believe that the blind application of methodologies designed for other purposes and circumstances is poor science.

Possible Solutions:

Here we have presented and clarified factors that impact in different ways alternative and traditional medicine as compared to biomedicine. To begin addressing many of these issues, we have designed a research program that will encompass the following issues:

- There is a commonality among various traditional systems of health, all of which describe a spiritual and "energy" basis for biological mechanisms. We propose to evaluate the physical and biological effects of nonmolecular interactions.

- There is great variety among alternative and traditional therapies, which include a variety of different health systems, some of which may be as complex as biomedicine itself. We propose to examine and evaluate the health benefits and economic impact of improved access to indigenous medicine by whole populations.
- Many traditional medical treatments are holistic and multifaceted. We are currently conducting an observational study on the effectiveness of a traditional health system approach to Irritable Bowel Syndrome (IBS). In this project, the practitioner will have no other constraints than to recruit suitable patients and accurately record the treatment.
- Each health system reflects the beliefs and philosophical systems of the culture from which it evolved. We are incorporating these considerations in Continuing Medical Education (CME) courses and other curricula designed for the healthcare professional. Furthermore, we plan to develop a school curriculum beginning in early childhood.
- Much of the healthcare system is driven by profit motives. We feel it is important to develop a project that will investigate and advance activities and outcomes other than consumption of medical goods as a basis for reimbursement.

You believe that such programs, if clearly and decisively coordinated, could have a profound impact on worldwide healthcare because the various facets of such programs touch upon the essence of the differences between traditional systems of health and biomedicine, not only from the medical, but also from cultural and values-based standpoints.

References

- Alternative, medical: disabled-world.com, Retrieved 26 March, 2019
- The effects of stimulant and tranquilizer placebos on healthy subjects in a real-life situation. Psychopharmacologia. 1965;7:444-52
- Types-of-complementary-and-alternative-medicine, wellness-and-prevention, health: hopkinsmedicine.org, Retrieved 14 April, 2019
- Assessing the effects of physicianpatient interactions on the outcomes of chronic disease. Med Care. 1989;27: S110-27
- Effective physician-patient communication and health outcomes: a review. CMAJ. 1995;152:1423-33

2

Whole Medical Systems and Alternative Medicine

Some common alternative practices which are followed across the globe include naturopathy, acupressure, Ayurveda, homeopathy, etc. This chapter discusses in detail the theories and methodologies related to these forms of alternative medicine.

Whole medical systems are built upon theories and practices that have evolved apart from, and earlier than, the conventional medical approach used in the United States. Whole medical systems that have developed in Western cultures include homeopathic medicine and naturopathic medicine. Examples of systems that have developed in non-Western cultures include Traditional Chinese Medicine and Ayurvedic Medicine.

Homeopathy

Homeopathy is an alternative medical system. It takes a different approach from conventional medicine in diagnosing, classifying, and treating medical problems. Key concepts of homeopathy include:

- Homeopathy seeks to stimulate the body's defense mechanisms and processes so as to prevent or treat illness.
- Treatment involves giving very small doses of substances (called remedies) that, according to homeopathy, would produce the same or similar symptoms of illness in healthy people if they were given in larger doses.
- Treatment in homeopathy is tailored to each person. Homeopathic practitioners select remedies according to a total picture of the patient, including not only symptoms but lifestyle, emotional and mental states, and other factors.

Most homeopathies in the United States are practiced along with another health care practice for which the practitioner is licensed, such as conventional medicine, naturopathy, chiropractic, dentistry, or acupuncture.

People report success with homeopathic treatments for psoriasis, including sulfur and nickel. Homeopathic remedies are usually so diluted that they will not cause major side effects. A consultation with someone trained in this practice will help guide the treatment and ensure your safety.

Naturopathy

Naturopathy, also called naturopathic medicine, focuses on supporting health rather than combating disease. The practice of naturopathy is based on six key principles:

- First do no harm: Naturopathic practitioners choose therapies with the intent to keep harmful side effects to a minimum and not suppress symptoms.
- Promote the healing power of nature.
- Treat the whole person: Practitioners believe a person's health is affected by many factors, such as physical, mental, emotional, genetic, environmental, and social ones. Practitioners consider all these factors when choosing therapies and tailor treatment to each patient.
- Treat the cause: Practitioners seek to identify and treat the causes of a disease or condition, rather than its symptoms. They believe that symptoms are signs that the body is trying to fight disease, adapt to it, or recover from it.
- Prevention is the best cure: Practitioners teach ways of living that they consider most healthy and most likely to prevent illness.
- The physician is a teacher: Practitioners consider it important to educate their patients in taking responsibility for their own health.

Traditional Chinese Medicine

Traditional Chinese medicine (TCM) is a whole medical system that originated in China. It is based on the concept that disease results from disruption in the flow of qi, vital energy, and imbalance in the forces of yin and yang. Practices such as herbs, meditation, massage, and acupuncture seek to aid healing by restoring the yin-yang balance and the flow of qi.

In the treatment of psoriasis, oral and topical herbal treatments are used. Psoriasis patients have used the following herbal topicals with some success: aloe, apple cider vinegar, capsaicin (a natural ingredient found in cayenne peppers), emu oil, evening primrose oil, oats, and tea tree oil.

Use caution with all herbals: Some make the skin more sensitive to ultraviolet light, while others may interact with other prescriptions or medications.

Acupuncture - Aims to restore and maintain health through the stimulation of specific points on the body using a variety of techniques. The acupuncture technique that has been most often studied scientifically involves penetrating the skin with thin, solid, metallic needles that are manipulated by the hands or by electrical stimulation. Qi can be unblocked, according to TCM, by using acupuncture at certain points on the body that connect with these meridians.

Reports from people with psoriasis or psoriatic arthritis are mixed: Some say acupuncture helps their disease while others report no effect. People who try acupuncture and improve say it takes many treatments. Acupuncture has few known side effects. According to the National Institutes of Health, acupuncture is an acceptable treatment for many pain conditions. Studies have shown that acupuncture helps relieve pain from fibromyalgia and osteoarthritis, so it may help relieve pain associated with psoriatic arthritis.

Ayurvedic Medicine (Ayurveda)

Ayurvedic medicine (also called Ayurveda) is one of the world's oldest medical systems. It originated in India and has evolved there over thousands of years. It aims to integrate and balance the body, mind, and spirit; thus, some view it as holistic, treating the body as a whole and not just the symptoms of an illness.

The aim of Ayurvedic medicine is to integrate and balance the body, mind, and spirit. This is believed to help prevent illness and promote wellness. Ayurvedic medicine uses a variety of products and techniques to cleanse the body and restore balance. Some of these products may be harmful if used improperly or without the direction of a trained practitioner. For example, some herbs can cause side effects or interact with conventional medicines.

Yoga – A practice from Ayurvedic medicine that combines breathing exercises, physical postures, and meditation. It is intended to calm the nervous system and balance the body, mind and spirit. There are various styles of yoga that people use for health purposes. They typically combine physical postures, breathing techniques, and meditation or relaxation. There are numerous schools of yoga. Hatha yoga, the most commonly practiced in the United States and Europe, emphasizes postures and breathing exercises. People use yoga for a variety of conditions and to achieve fitness and relaxation. Yoga has also been used in Traditional Chinese medicine and is also considered a Mind-Body medicine technique.

Yoga can help bring stress under control. Some people with psoriatic arthritis anecdotally report that yoga can help ease pain and improve range of motion.

Acupressure

Acupressure has been practiced in China for more than 2000 years, but is only recently beginning to gain acceptance by Western medical practitioners as a legitimate means of treating symptoms of illness. It is a very popular complementary therapy at present and plays an important role in multidisciplinary approach to the treatment and management of various symptoms.

This therapy is a means of manipulating the same acupoints as used in acupuncture, but without the use of neddles. Acupressure is a noninvasive, safe and effective massage technique that employes pressure and massage to acupoints in order to stimulate the balance of life energy that in term promotes health and comfort. The therapy can be easily taught to patients so that they can manage fatigue, and decrease advers health outcomes to improve their quality of life.

The purposes of acupressure are to regulate and balance the body energy or Chi, and further to maintain health, prevent illness or enhance health. This energy referred to as Chi. Chi flows through the 12 major energy pathways called meridians, each linked to specific internal organs system and 365-2000 acupoints. Chi energy also regulate spiritual, emotional, mental and physical health.

Acupressure therapy is applied with the fingers on the acupoints and the stimulation lines or meridians of the body surface. The meridians start at the finger tips, connect to the brain, and than connect to the organ associated with the specific meridian.

These meridians can become blocked or slowed. Through applying pressure (acupressure) into one or more of these acupoints, imbalances can be corrected by stimulating or easing energy flow.

Each meridian is classified according to the specific organ to which it is associated. For example, the heart meridian is connected to the heart; the lung meridian is connected to the lungs.

Application of Acupressure

Acupressure is a type of stimulation of the body's acupuncture points by applying pressure using hands, fingers, palms, elbows, knees, thumbs or acustimulations bands more commonly known as Sea-Bands (Relief Bands or Wrist Bands). Sea –bands are bands or elasticated fabric with a small round plastic button inside the band. They are designed to be worn on both wrists.

The most commonly two acupoints used in acupressure are Pericardium 6 (P6 or Neiguaun) and Stomach 36 (ST36 or Zusanli). Pericardium 6 is situated bilaterally on the pericardium meridian. This is located on the anterior surface of the forearm, approximately three finger widths from the first wrist crease. The ST36 point is located bilaterally on the stomach meridian approximately for finger widths below the knee and one finger width lateral to the tibia.

Pressure on the Neiguan point, also called P6 or pericardial median, rebalances the energy life force or Chi when balance between the negative and positive energies (the Yin and the Yang) is achieved. According to the theory of Yin and Yang, life takes place in the alternating rhythm of Yin and Yang.

Acupressure should never be applied directly to wounds, bruises or sprains since strong finger pressure may increase pain and tissue damage. Hovewer, you can gently press points near the site of injury to increase circulation and release muscular tension.

The Effects of Acupressure

There are a number of theories as to how acupressure works. First, acuppressure alters brain chemistry by affecting the release of neurotransmitters and neurohormones. Second, it activates opioid systems, which is believed to account for the well – proven effects of these methods on pain. Third, it speeds up the transmission of electromagnetic signals that may activate the flow of endorphins and monuamines, and in turn, reduce levels of agitation and nausea.

A cupressure acts to dilate capillaries and accelerate (enhance) blood circulation locally; promote the flow of venous blood and lymphatic flood back to the hearth; increase erythrocyte counts and the level of leucocytes in the blood; strenghthen an individual's immunity; promote supple joint; stimulate large areas of nerve fiber by touch, pressing and rubbing to further activate substantia gelatinosa and influence the activities of T-cells that lead to less stimulation of cerebrum by pain and alleviate individual's pain; and finally, stimulate the arcuate nucleus of the thalamus to secrete endorphins.

The Benefits of Acupressure

Acupressure restores the body's energy flow and facilitates the healing process. It also improves blood flow and circulation so that oxygen can be carried more effectively to all parts of the body, increases energy and boosts the immune system.

Acupressure has been found to alleviate lower back pain, headaches, osteoarthritis pain, neck pain, musculoskeletal pain, menstrual pain, dental pain, fibromyalgia pain, pain before and after surgery, stomach pain and indigestion, other conditions with chronic pain.

Acupressure has been used to improve the quality of sleep and to reduce fatigue, to prevent postoperative and chemotherapy induced nausea and vomiting. It also alleviate the depression symptoms in hemodialysis patients.

Acupressure therapy can decrease sympathetic stimulation, promote relaxation and improve perceived symptoms of dyspnoea, anxiety and reduce physiological indicators of heart rates and respiratory rates in patients with chronic obstructive pulmonary diease who are using prolonged mechanical ventilation.

Acupuncture

Acupuncture is based on the idea that living beings have an inner energy, known as Qi (pronounced chee), and it is the flow of this inner energy that sustains them. According to traditional Chinese medical philosophy, balanced Qi is vital to optimal health; illness and disease are caused by the imbalance or interruption in the flow of Qi. Although acupuncture was developed for prevention of illness, it is useful in managing disease symptoms by reintroducing balanced flow of Qi, its main focus.

Jesuit missionaries introduced acupuncture to Europe in the 17th century, when they returned from China. The Jesuits were active in disseminating the idea and practice of acupuncture throughout Europe. In addition, traveling physicians helped pioneer acupuncture use in Europe.

In the United States, acupuncture gained public and professional attention in 1971.

Working of Accupuncture

Anatomically, acupuncture points have been reported to correspond to cutaneous areas of high electrical conductivity and distinct histologic differences compared with adjacent tissue. There are many theories that may explain how acupuncture works.

Gate Control Theory of Pain

This theory postulates that specific nerve fibers transmit a pain signal to the brain via the spinal cord, and input of other nerve fibers can inhibit the pain signal transmission. Acupuncture is thought to stimulate inhibitory nerve fibers for a short period, thus reducing transmission of the pain signal to the brain.

Endorphin Model

During the 1970s, researchers isolated endogenous endorphins in the central nervous system. Clinical studies reported that inserting acupuncture needles into specific acupuncture points triggered the production of endorphins in cerebrospinal fluid after patients underwent acupuncture treatments. The pain-alleviating effects of acupuncture were reduced when naloxone was used to pretreat the patient, which may indicate that acupuncture-induced analgesia may be partly mediated through endogenous opioids.

Recent research has found that traditional Chinese medicine acupuncture therapy has a direct effect in the up-regulation of m-opioid receptor binding availability in the central nervous system compared with placebo (sham) acupuncture. This finding may help explain some of the analgesic effects seen with acupuncture therapy.

Neurotransmitter Model

Research in animals has found that acupuncture can modulate serotonin, norepinephrine, and neurons that transmit or secrete g-aminobutyric acid. It is postulated that through the neurotransmitter model, acupuncture can be efficacious for treatment of depression, anxiety, and addiction.

Other Theories

Other theories postulate that acupuncture indirectly influences the autonomic system. Acupuncture treatment can affect respiration, heart rate, blood pressure, circulation, and immune function. Research indicates the increased electrical conductivity of tissues along acupuncture meridians. This result suggests that manipulation of the acupuncture meridians with needles may modulate the transmission of certain signals within the body. The current scientific theories provide a basis for stating that acupuncture has an effect on the nervous system, but its effects cannot be explained with a single mechanism.

Is Acupuncture Safe?

Modern acupuncture needles are thin and flexible and are made of solid surgical stainless steel. Unlike hypodermic needles, acupuncture needles are finely tapered, allowing them to slide smoothly into the skin. Certain acupuncture needles are thinner than the average strand of human hair.

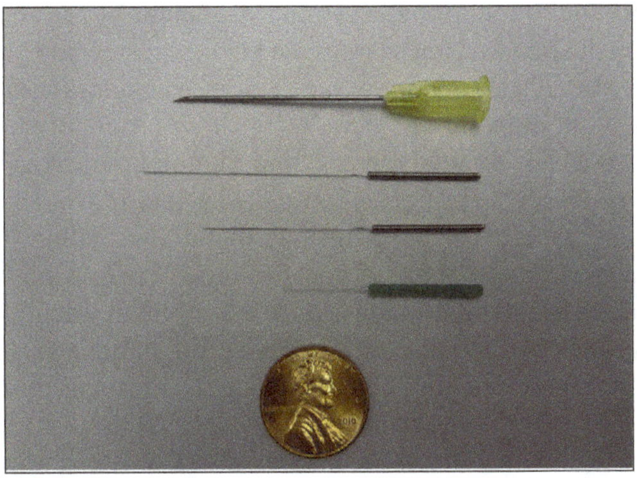

Comparison of acupuncture needles with a 20-gauge hypodermic needle. Coin shown for indication of needle sizes.

Acupuncture in the developed parts of the world involves single-use, disposable needles packaged and sealed by the manufacturer in sterile conditions. Although case reports have highlighted major adverse events, such as organ puncture, infections, and bleeding complications, more recent, larger cohort studies using universal precautions have not found a significant complication rate. In a 2001 study of more than 34,000 acupuncture treatments in the United Kingdom, no serious adverse events (eg, hospitalization, permanent disability, or death) were reported in relation to acupuncture therapy, and the rate of underlying minor adverse events (eg, nausea, fainting, prolonged aggravation of existing symptoms, and psychological or emotional reaction) was reported to be between 0 and 1.1 per 10,000 treatments. Acupuncture involves puncturing the skin, and therefore slight bruising, bleeding, or soreness at the acupuncture site may occur because of needle penetration through capillaries. More serious adverse effects, such as a vasovagal response with a decrease in blood pressure and syncope, have been reported. Infections may occur at the needle site from the use of nonsterile needles. When herbs are burned too close to the skin, burn injuries can result around the needle site. Most patients communicate a sense of relaxation and well-being after a treatment.

Acupuncture is generally considered safe for persons with bleeding disorders or taking anticoagulants. However, it is important for the patient to advise the practitioner of these facts so the practitioner can use vigilance in selecting insertion points. Acupuncture during pregnancy is a matter of continued debate. Certain acupuncture points are contraindicated because they may induce uterine contractions and premature labor.

Ayurvedic Medicine

India is known for its traditional medicinal systems— Ayurveda, Siddha, and Unani. Medical systems are found mentioned even in the ancient Vedas and other scriptures. The Ayurvedic concept appeared and developed between 2500 and 500 BC in India.The literal meaning of Ayurveda is "science of life," because ancient Indian system of health care focused on views of man and his illness. It has been pointed out that the positive health means metabolically wellbalanced human beings. Ayurveda is also called the "science of longevity" because it offers a complete system to live a long healthy life. It offers programs to rejuvenate the body through diet and nutrition. It offers treatment methods to cure many common diseases such as food allergies, which have few modern treatments. However, one should be aware that Ayurvedic nutrition is not a "magic bullet" system but requires the full participation of the patient to succeed. It is an interactive system that is user-friendly and educational. It teaches the patient to become responsible and self-empowered. Ayurveda is not a nutritional system for those seeking an escape or excuse to further abuse their body or mind. It is a system for empowerment, a system of freedom, and long life.

Food is the major source for serving the nutritional needs, but with growing modernization some traditional methods are being given up. Hence, the modern food habits are affecting the balanced nutrition. There is an ever widening gap in nutrient intake due to which normal life is no longer normal. However, affluence of working population with changing lifestyles and reducing affordability of sick care, in terms of time and money involved, are some of the forces that are presently driving people towards thinking about their wellness.

Medicinal Plants used in Alternative/Traditional Medicines

Alternative medicines are being used by about 60 percent of the world's population. These medicines are not only used by the rural masses for their primary health care in developing countries but are also used in developed countries where modern medicines dominate. The Indian subcontinent is a vast repository of medicinal plants that are used in traditional medical treatments. The alternative medicines in the traditional systems are derived from herbs, minerals, and organic matter, while for the preparation of herbal drugs only medicinal plants are used. Use of plants as a source of medicine has been an ancient practice and is an important component of the health care system in India. In India, about 70 percent of rural population depends on the traditional Ayurvedic system of medicine. Most healers/practitioners of the traditional systems of medicine prepare formulations by their own recipes and dispense to the patients. In the Western countries, approximately 40 per cent of people are using the herbal medicine for mmonly seek conventional carthe treatment of various diseases. This interest in traditional medicines is growing rapidly due to the attention being given to it by the governmental agencies and different NGO's comprising of general public and researchers as well as the increased side effects, adverse drug reactions, and cost factor of the modern medicines.

Table: Impact of modern food concept in required nutrition.

Nutrients	Intake by traditional ways	Intake by modern ways	Effect on nutrient intake
Water soluble vitamins (vitamins B and C) and minerals	Vegetables used for cooking were/are fresh.	Freezing and packaging of the cut vegetables.	Loss of ascorbic acid, water soluble vitamins, and minerals.
Proteins, minerals, and vitamin B complex	Manual processing of cereals, without polishing.	Milling and polishing of Cereals.	Reduces protein, minerals, and vitamin B complex.
Calcium, iron, thiamine, and niacin	Fresh grinding at home.	Heavy milling and poor storage conditions.	Loss of calcium, iron, thiamin, and Niacin.
Iron	Cooking in iron pot.	Food generally cooked in cookware like non-stick and Teflon-coated utensils.	The benefit of organic iron from the conventional iron pot is not obtained by using modern cookware.
Copper	Storing of water and cooking use of copper vessels.	Stainless steel utensils and plastic wares.	Copper required in minor amount which is not gained from modern utensils used today. Deficiency is known to cause chronic diarrhea, malabsorption problems, and reduce immunity. Use of plastic containers is also harmful.

India is the largest producer of medicinal plants. There are currently about 250,000 registered medical practitioners of the Ayurvedic system, as compared to about 700,000 of the modern medicine. In India, around 20,000 medicinal plants have been recorded; however, traditional practitioners use only 7,000–7,500 plants for curing different diseases. The proportion of use of plants in the different Indian systems of medicine is Ayurveda 2000, Siddha 1300, Unani 1000, Homeopathy 800, Tibetan 500, Modern 200, and folk 4500. In India, around 25,000 effective plant-based formulations are used in traditional and folk medicine. More than 1.5 million practitioners are using the traditional medicinal system for health care in India. It is estimated that more than 7800 manufacturing units are involved in the production of natural health products and traditional plant-based formulations in India, which requires more than 2000 tons of medicinal plant raw material annually. More than 1500 herbals are sold as dietary supplements or ethnic traditional medicines.

Alternative medicines are being used by those people who do not use or cannot be helped by conventional medicinal system.

Expanding Complementary and Alternative (CAM) Approaches

More than 80 percent of people in developing countries cannot afford the most basic medical procedures, drugs, and vaccines. Among wealthier populations in both developed and developing countries, complementary and alternative practices are popular although proof of their safety and effectiveness is modest. Evidence-based research in Ayurveda is receiving larger acceptance in India and abroad. The National Center for Complementary and Alternative Medicine has been inaugurated as the United States Federal Government's lead agency for scientific research in this arena of medicine. Its mission is to explore complementary and alternative healing practices in the context of rigorous science, support sophisticated research, train researchers, disseminate information to the public on the modalities that work, and explain the scientific rationale underlying discoveries. The center is committed to explore and fund all such therapies for which there is sufficient preliminary data, compelling public health need and ethical justifications.

Complementary and alternative practices are adjuncts or alternatives to Western medical approaches. Economic factors influence user behavior. Although social, cultural, and medical reasons account for most of the appeal of traditional approaches, economic factors also play a role. It is assumed that users of these approaches choose them because they are cheaper than conventional therapies or systems. However, several studies have found that CAM approaches cost the same or more than conventional treatments for the same conditions; thus, people seek them out for reasons other than cost. At least one study showed that financial factors ranked behind such reasons as confidence in the treatment, ease of access, and convenience, in the choice of a traditional healer. Another common misconception is that the poor are more likely to use traditional medicine, but this is not always true. Nowadays people seek CAM techniques because they believe the side effects will be lower. In both developed and developing countries, users of complementary methods also commonly seek conventional care.

Ayurveda has the distinction of being the "oldest medical system known to man and the oldest and most comprehensive spiritual teachings in the world". Ayurveda is based on the principle of maintaining a balance between the interrelated relationships within the body and mind. It helps the patient to understand the benefits of knowing their body and mind and to live in intimate relationship with nature. Ayurvedic literature has remedies for age-related diseases like memory loss, osteoporosis, diabetic wounds, etc. for which no efficient medicine is available in modern therapy. Ayurvedic formulations should be standardized on the basis of active principle or major compound(s) along with fingerprints. Ayurveda is a holistic system of medical science and is the oldest healing science which is almost 5000 years old. Ayurveda contains two Sanskrit words: Ayu which means life or lifespan and Veda meaning knowledge. Thus, Ayurveda means "the science of life." This system of medicine was shaped in the ancient lands of India. Hindu Vedas consider Ayurveda as a gift of Gods to mankind which was communicated to the saints and sages of India through deep meditation. Veda Vyasa, one of the greatest sages of India is considered to have written the Vedas for the first time. Ayurveda, recognized as new age medicine now, represents the science of life and longevity originating in the Vedic tradition of India. Based on the principle of eternal life, this medical system has a vast body of knowledge covering eight branches. Its major premise involves the symbiosis of mind, body and spirit. Any imbalance in this synthesis results in physical ailments. This ancient Indian science of healing seeks to re-establish the harmony between the body and its habitat by creating the optimum health environment.

The entire science of ayurveda is based on the 'Five Great Elements' (Panchabhuta) theory. These five elements are earth (prithvi), water (jal), fire (agni or tej), air (vayu) and ether or space (akash). Ayurveda comprehends body, mind and spirit likewise and has specific methods for working on each. It divides the constitution of people into three humoral categories-Vata (ether/air), Pitta (fire) and Kapha (water/earth). Vata rules mental mobility. Pitta or fire, governs digestion and assimilation on all levels from food to ideas and Kapha or water, governs form and substance and is responsible for weight, cohesion and stability. According to the concept of good management, ayurveda insists that the 'Fault' or Dosha, the 'Tissue' or Dhatu and the 'Impurity' or Mala should be in harmony with each other, with all the components properly balanced. These are basically therapeutic measures taken either to prevent diseases or cure them. Thus, ayurvedic procedures are done either to detoxify the body or as a prelude to strengthening the immune system. Even today ayurvedic medicine maintains its holistic approach to health and treatment of diseases. The branches of modern ayurveda include:

- Principles of preventive healthcare for the entire family.
- Treatment of addictions.

- Purification and rejuvenation treatments.
- The ayurvedic approach to diet and weight loss.
- Musculoskeletal system treatments.
- Promotion of self-healing and resistance to disease.
- Male and female infertility.
- Beauty and cosmetic treatments for men and women.
- Ayurveda objective is to help the healthy person to maintain good health and the diseased person to regain good health. The practice of Ayurveda is designed to promote human happiness at physical, mental and spiritual level. By the proper balance of all vital energies in the body, the processes of physical deterioration and disease can be reduced. This is accomplished through proper eating, thinking and living habits as well as the use of herbal remedies to treat illness.
- In Ayurveda one is in good health when our inner and internal environment is in balance.
- The Vata, Pitta and Kapha dosha are in balance.
- Agni (the digestive fire) is balanced.
- Dhatus (the 7 body tissues) are functioning normally.
- Mala (the waste products) are produced and eliminated normally.
- The Mana, Indriya and Atma (mind, senses and consciousness) are working in blissful harmony.

Ayurvedic Medicine

Ayurvedic medicine (also called Ayurveda) is one of the world's oldest medical systems. It originated in India and has evolved there over thousands of years. In the United States, Ayurvedic medicine is considered complementary and alternative medicine (CAM)—more specifically, a CAM whole medical system. Many therapies used in Ayurvedic medicine are also used on their own as CAM—for example, herbs, massage, and specialized diets. The aim of Ayurvedic medicine is to integrate and balance the body, mind, and spirit. This is believed to help prevent illness and promote wellness. Ayurvedic medicine uses a variety of products and techniques to cleanse the body and restore balance. Some of these products may be harmful if used improperly or without the direction of a trained practitioner. For example, some herbs can cause side effects or interact with conventional medicines.

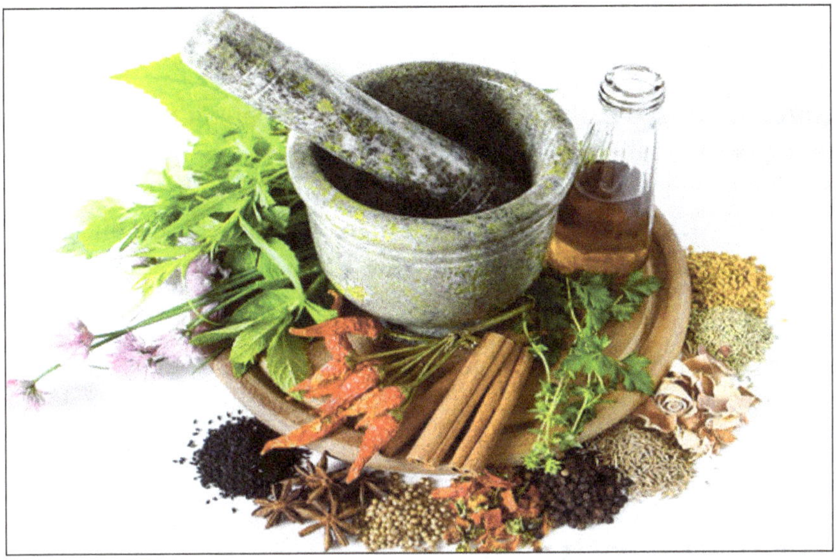

Ingredients used in Ayurvedic Medicine.

Ayurvedic medicine also treats specific physical and mental health problems. A chief aim of Ayurvedic practices is to cleanse the body of substances that can cause disease, thus helping to re-establish harmony and balance.

Key Foundations of Ayurveda

Ayurvedic medicines have several key foundations thatpertain to health and disease. These concepts have to do with universal interconnectedness, the body's constitution *(prakriti),* and life forces *(doshas).*

Interconnectedness

Ideas about the relationships among people, their health, and the universe form the basis for how Ayurvedic practitioners think about problems that affect health. Ayurvedic medicine holds that:

- All things in the universe (both living and nonliving) are joined together.
- Every human being contains elements that can be found in the universe.
- Health will be good if one's mind and body are in harmony, and one's interaction with the universe is natural and wholesome.
- Disease arises when a person is out of harmony with the universe. Disruptions can be physical, emotional, spiritual, or a combination of these.

Constitution (Prakriti)

Ayurvedic medicine also has specific beliefs about the body's constitution. Constitution refers to a person's general health, the likelihood of becoming out of balance, and the ability to resist and recover from disease or other health problems.

The constitution is called the *prakriti*. The *prakriti* is a person's unique combination of physical and psychological characteristics and the way the body functions to maintain health. It is influenced by such factors as digestion and how the body deals with waste products. The *prakriti* is believed to be unchanged over a person's lifetime.

Life Forces (Doshas)

Important characteristics of the *prakriti* are the three life forces or energies called *doshas,* which control the activities of the body. A person's chances of developing certain types of diseases are thought to be related to the way *doshas* are balanced, the state of the physical body, and mental or lifestyle factors.

Function of Ayurvedic Medicine

Ayurveda holds specific belief about general health and physical body. General quality of health is referred to as 'prakriti' or constitution in ayurveda. Praktiti consist three energies namely, vata, pitta and kapha.

- Pitta is made up of fire and water.
- Vata is made up of space and air.
- Kapha is made of water and earth.

Ayurvedic medicine helps to balance these doshas and increase body's ability to resist and recover from diseases.

Benefits of Ayurvedic Medicines

- Ayurvedic medicine aims at maintaining and restoring body's own capability to have balance and fight with ailments.
- Ayurvedic medicines can be safely used with other conventional medicines.
- They are non-toxic and non-invasive.
- Ayurvedic medicines are widely used to treat several physical as well as psychological conditions. Arthritis, obesity, hypertension, heart disease, nervous disorder, colds, colitis, constipation, obesity, skin problem, ulcer, acne, allergies, asthma, anxiety, chronic fatigue syndrome, depression, diabetes, flu and immune problems.
- Ayurvedic practitioners claim that with ayurvedic medicines one can easily get relieve from stress and problem in metabolism.

- Since Ayurvedic medicines have natural ingredients, they do not have any side effects. These medicines make the person's body and mind disease free.

Homeopathy

Homeopathy is an effective and scientific system of healing that assists the natural tendency of the body to heal itself. It recognizes that all symptoms of ill health are expressions of disharmony within the whole person and that it is the individual person who needs treatment, not the disease. The homeopathic principles constitute a unified hypothesis whose validity is tested empirically: cured patients confirm the hypothesis. Homeopathic medicines are prepared in a pharmacy or a laboratory, using a technique subject to precise and clearly stated controls. The preparation and administration of homeopathic medicines does not involve mysterious processes.

Homeopathy is an increasingly popular alternative system of medicine whose basic philosophy is viewed skeptically by the orthodox medical profession because it is difficult to understand within accepted scientific theories. Its success with patients, however, has led to its continual growth and development over the past 200 years, culminating in a resurgence in recent years partly owing to increasing dissatisfaction with the side effects of modern medicines.

Homeopathy is based on the principles of similars. The standard medical assumption is this: if the body produces a symptom, the appropriate treatment is an antidote, or opposite medicine, whose purpose is to overcome that symptom. For example, a conventional doctor will treat constipation with a laxative, which produces diarrhea. The premise of the law of similars is this: any substance that can cause symptoms of disease in a healthy person can cure a sick person who manifests a similar symptom profile. A homeopathic practitioner treats constipation by giving a homeopathic medicine that has produced symptoms of constipation in a healthy person.

Treating "like with like" was described by Hippocrates in the 5th century BC; the "father of medicine," and people throughout the world have employed this principle of healing with "similars" for many hundreds of years. It was the German doctor Samuel Hahnemann, however, who discovered this basic approach through an experiment he conducted on himself, in an attempt to understand how medicines worked. Questioning the basis for treating malaria with quinine, Hahnemann ingested Cinchona bark (from which quinine is derived) in order to find out how it might affect a healthy person. After a number of days, he started to experience symptoms of fever (typical of malaria), which cleared up once he stopped taking the medicine.

Hahnemann next experimented with Cinchona bark on family and friends, with similar results. This led him to experiment with many other substances in order to discover what symptoms of illness they could produce in healthy individuals. He called these tests provings and meticulously recorded individual reactions as well as any common themes or patterns of illness produced by each substance–including sensations and feelings. These provings formed the basis of a new system of healing Hahnemann called homeopathy, from the Greek homo- ios (similar) and pathos (suffering or disease), in order to differentiate it from orthodox medicine, which he called "allopathy," meaning "opposite suffering".

Hahnemann then used the "symptom pictures" he assembled as the basis for his prescriptions. He gave a single medicine at a time, as opposed to the medical practice of his time, which involved mixtures containing many medicines. His departure from "accepted" medical practice attracted much derision, especially from the apothecaries, but the successes he achieved with patients verified his theory, and he continued to develop his system.

Hahnemann experimented with diluting his medicines to minimize side effects but found that simple dilution (with stirring) caused the medicine to lose its efficacy altogether, so he developed a new method of dilution whereby he diluted the substance in carefully measured steps, shaking it vigorously in between each dilution. This shaking he called "succussion" and the resultant liquid a "potentized remedy." He found that this new remedy lacked side effects and had a stronger curative.

reaction. In fact, he discovered that the more he diluted and succussed a substance the stronger it became. This dilution-and-potency issue has become "one of the main areas of controversy in the homeopathic system".

This process of dilution consistently incurred scepticism from the medical establishment which could not explain, and therefore could not accept, how anything so dilute could have an effect. Despite such opposition, homeopathy survived because it worked, and patients who were helped spread the word. Some of those patients were doctors and many of them, having experienced the gentle yet effective healing power of homeopathy themselves, then trained under Hahnemann and took his teachings out into the world, to South and North America, India and Europe.

The Principles

Simillimum

The homeopathic remedy is selected on the basis that it causes similar symptoms in a healthy person, as documented in experiments that are called provings. This remedy is known as the simillimum.

Minimum Dose

Dilution with succussion releases the strength or "potency" of any substance and makes it a more effective medicine while eliminating potential side effects. Homeopathic medicines are made from a wide variety of substances—animal, vegetable, and mineral. Because a homeopathic remedy is diluted beyond the point where there is anything measurable of the original substance— at a molecular level—absolutely anything can be used, including some which are toxic at a material dose, such as acids and snake venoms.

The starting remedy—a tincture or mother tincture— is made by steeping soluble substances in alcohol and then straining them. Insoluble substances are ground for several hours with a pestle and mortar until they are rendered soluble. This process, called trituration, is used for metals and other substances that do not dissolve easily in order to prepare them for dilution and succussion.

There are two scales for diluting substances: the decimal and the centesimal. For the decimal scale, one tenth of the tincture is added to nine tenths alcohol and shaken vigorously; this first dilution is called a 1X. The number of a homeopathic remedy reflects the number of times it has been diluted and succussed: for example, Sulphur 6X has been diluted and succussed six times.

The centesimal scale is diluted using one part in a hundred of the tincture and the letter C is added after the number. Paradoxically, a 6X is called a low potency and 20 °C a high potency; the greater the dilution, the greater the potency, the stronger the curative potential of the medicine.

The most commonly used potency in the decimal scale is the 6X, although the 9X, 12X, 24X, and 30X are used by some. In the centesimal scale, those potencies most commonly used are the 6 °C, 12 °C, 3 °C, and 20 °C.

Single Remedy

Remedies are tested, or proven, one at a time and prescribed on an individual basis. Combination remedies (including several remedies that are strongly indicated in a particular disease) are widely available in this country, although results are likely to be disappointing if the single remedy a person needs is not included in a particular mixture.

Whole Person

Every human being should be viewed as a unique individual, whole and complete, functioning as a totality in relation to the surrounding environment; in this context, the only way to cure illness is to increase the health of the afflicted person. Based on this philosophy, alternative treatments look at the disease within the "whole person context." They take into account the person who has become ill, and their treatment is designed to stimulate that person's own self-healing abilities. Alternative health care practitioners believe it is important to exploreboth how a person has become ill, as well as the known stressors in their lives, especially those that have led up to illness and will take these into account when planning a course of treatment. Many people find this a relief and are grateful to be treated as a whole rather than having to separate themselves into "parts" to be handed over to a host of "experts."

Vital Force

The human organism has a unique relationship with its environment, which biologists refer to as "homeostasis." As such, a healthy living being is self-regulating, with an innate (protective) tendency to maintain its equilibrium and compensate for disruptive changes. Hahnemann believed that an energetic substance, independent of physical and chemical forces, exists and that this "vital force" gives life and is absent at death. It is also known as chi or prana by Eastern medical practitioners. This vital force acts in predictable ways and operates both in sickness and in health, by producing coping mechanisms to counteract stressors. Disease is the body's way of coping with stress. Homeopaths credit this balancing mechanism for the maintenance of health, provided that the stresses on the mind and body are neither too prolonged nor too great.

Susceptibility and Constitutional Treatment

Susceptibility is simply the degree to which a person is vulnerable to an outside influence. Not everyone who goes for a walk in a cold wind will be affected, but some are "susceptible." Their predisposition is due to an underlying constitutional weakness, which is either inherited or due to past and/or current stress (mental, emotional, or physical).

Many people consult a homeopath to receive "constitutional treatment" for chronic complaints that have not been alleviated through other forms of treatment. The value of such treatment is that it boosts the weak constitution and decreases its susceptibility to disease. This type of intervention requires specialized education and training.

How Does Homeopathy Work?

Although homeopathy has been compared to vaccination, they are very different practices. Vaccines stimulate the immune system directly to produce specific antibodies to a particular disease. They are tested on animals and then on humans to verify their safety; even then side effects are common. Most vaccines are introduced directly into the bloodstream, bypassing the body's natural defense system and stimulating it in a way that is not fully understood.

Homeopathic medicines are administered orally in safe, diluted, and succussed doses; they are tested on healthy humans (not on animals), and when used correctly have no side effects. They work on an individual's energy patterns, by stimulating the immune system generally.

Naturopathy

Many of the philosophical principles that underpin naturopathic practice can be traced to the teachings of Stoicism in ancient Greece and the practice of medicine in the Hippocratic schools. In addition to these ancient roots, naturopathic practice emerged from an amalgamation of the philosophy, techniques, science and principles that typified the alternative healing systems of the eighteenth and nineteenth centuries, particularly those related to vitalism. These alternative approaches tended to focus both on health promotion and on health-care regimes that supported the patient's innate healing processes.

Some of the founding influences that defined naturopathic philosophy and practice include:

- The hydrotherapy techniques of Vincent Priessnitz and Father Sebastian Kneipp in Europe, and John Harvey Kellogg in North America;
- The Thomsonian method of Samuel Thomson that foreshadowed physiomedicalism, from which some forms of modern phytotherapy emerged;
- The nature cure methods of Dr Louis Kuhne, Dr Arnold Rickli, and Dr Henry Lindlahr that emphasized healthy lifestyles, sunlight and fresh air, vegetarianism and detoxification;
- Homeopathy, derived by Christian Friedrich Samuel Hahnemann;
- The Eclectic school of medicine of Dr Wooster Beach, which employed botanical medicines;
- The philosophy of vitalism, which maintained that the body has an innate intelligence that strives constantly for health, so that the practitioner's role is to assist these efforts by cooperating with the healing powers of nature active within the body; schools of manipulative therapies, such as osteopathy, developed by Dr Andrew Taylor Still, and chiropractic, developed by Daniel David Palmer.

In Europe, the naturopathic approach to health care tended to evolve from the hydrotherapy and nature cure practices that had been developed by Priessnitz, Kneipp, Kuhne and Rickli. In North America, Dr Benedict Lust is described as establishing naturopathy in 1902, deriving it from nature cure. Naturopathy has been regulated in various regions of Europe and North America since the 1920s. The practice of naturopathy can vary widely, depending on the history of its evolution, the legislation affecting its practice, and the demands of the public for traditional medicine and complementary and alternative medicine (TM/CAM) in the relevant jurisdiction.

From the mid-1960s into the 1980s, naturopathy enjoyed a renaissance as the public in many parts of the world became disenchanted with so-called "western" medical practices and more interested in holistic health-care practices that emphasize healthy lifestyles as well as health promotion and disease prevention. Various modalities exist. As universities began to emphasize the need for credible research and scientific validation in every discipline and the demand for "evidence-based medicine" continued to grow, naturopathic practitioners continued their support for high academic standards and sound curricula to pursue the scientific confirmation of naturopathic methods. For instance, an international council for the accreditation of naturopathic colleges was established in North America as well as a central agency to examine the graduates of naturopathic colleges. These efforts at formalizing and universalizing standards of naturopathic education and practice established new benchmarks and intensified discussion concerning the identity of the profession.

The principles that inform naturopathy can be summarized as follows:

- "First, do no harm".
- Act in cooperation with the healing power of nature.
- Seek, identify and treat the fundamental cause of the illness.
- Treat the whole person using individualized treatment.
- Teach the principles of healthy living and preventive health care.

While the emphasis placed on these principles can vary within naturopathy, each version generally captures the same underlying philosophy and goals.

First, Do No Harm

Although a seemingly obvious statement that would be echoed by any healthcare practitioner, the dictum attributed to the classical physician Hippocrates, that physicians should "do no harm" to their patients, has specific resonance in naturopathy. As in most health-care professions, investigative methods and therapeutic modalities that do the least harm to the patient are preferred. When other health-care approaches are required because of the patient's illness, naturopathic practitioners are trained to recognize this situation and to refer patients to those who can provide the needed care.

Act in Cooperation with the Healing Power of Nature

The Stoics of ancient Greece believed that there was an animating principle, logos, that acted as a vital force to order the universe. If humans used their rational abilities to bring their behaviour into harmony with this order, they would flourish. Naturopathy, adopting this Stoic philosophy, recognizes that the same power that made the body – i.e. an innate intelligence active both in the universe and within the human body – would also heal the body unless prevented from doing so. By working with this healing power of nature – i.e. working with the vis medicatrix naturae of the patient – rather than trying to impose a treatment without regard for the person's own intrinsic ability to heal, the naturopathic practitioner seeks to assist the body, mind and spirit of the patient to bring about the desired healing.

Seek, Identify and Treat the Fundamental Cause of the Illness

For every problem, there is a cause. Naturopathic practitioners are more interested in seeking, identifying and treating the cause than in treating the symptoms of illness. They argue that if the symptom of a disease is temporarily eliminated or suppressed but the underlying cause is neglected, then the problem will simply return, or could even worsen in the interim. The cause of illness must be identified and eliminated if true healing is to occur. This often requires a thorough examination of the patient's lifestyle, diet and vital force.

Treat the Whole Person Using Individualized Treatment

Naturopathic practitioners work with a holistic understanding of human health. They recognize that humans are most likely to experience optimal health when their physical, psychological, spiritual and environmental dimensions are holistically integrated. People who exhibit integrated health are better able to realize their goals and actualize their potential. They are more likely to be in harmony within themselves, with others and with their environment. Because each person is different, the naturopathic practitioner must individualize treatments to meet the unique needs of each patient.

Teach the Principles of Healthy Living and Preventive Health Care

Naturopathic practitioners teach the principles of healthy living and preventive health care. They teach patients the causes of illnesses so that the patients are better able to avoid recurrences. Furthermore, patients should be involved in the therapeutic process so that they can engage in their own recovery and learn to take responsibility for their future health. This cooperative approach between the practitioner and patient has been shown to empower the patient, which provides further benefit. It is also more likely to engender a positive attitude in the patient, which is believed to improve the chances of optimal recovery.

References

- Whole-systems, alternative, treatments, about-psoriasis: psoriasis.org, Retrieved 10 August, 2019
- "Radical scavenging and ironchelating activities of some greens used as traditional dishes in

Mediterranean diet," International Journal of Food Sciences and Nutrition, vol. 55, no. 1, pp. 67–74, 2004

- "Indian herbal drug for general healthcare: an overview," The Internet Journal of Alternative Medicine, vol. 6, no. 1, p. 3, 2008
- Importance-of-ayurvedic-medicine-in-modern-lifestyle-A-keynote-review-study-324783389: researchgate.net, Retrieved 17 June, 2019
- "Postnatal development and reproductive performance of F1 progeny exposed in utero to an ayurvedic contraceptive: Pippaliyadi yoga," Journal of Ethnopharmacology, vol. 109, no. 3, pp. 406–411, 2007

3

Mind-body Medicines

Mind-body medicine refers to a system of medicine which seeks to understand the effect of emotions and mind on the physical health of an organism. The topics elaborated in this chapter such as meditation and biofeedback therapy will help in gaining a better perspective about mind-body medicine.

There was a time not long ago when Western medicine believed that health depended solely upon the physical mechanisms of the body. That is, a person is made up only of physical and chemical reactions that can be measured and manipulated scientifically. The notion that the mind and body live in separate compartments, so to speak, goes back to certain philosophers of classical antiquity. This concept of mind/body separation was also present in such religious groups as the Gnostics and some sects on the fringes of medieval Christianity. The scientific version of this split between mind and body is generally traced back to the seventeenth-century French philosopher Rene Descartes, whose thinking aided the development of science. It has taken a lot of time and research, three centuries after Descartes, for mainstream medicine to begin to accept that the mind plays a major role in health and disease.

The idea that the mind and body interact is not new, however. It can be traced to the Wisdom literature in the Old Testament and to Hippocrates, the father of Western medicine. The ancient Hebrews attributed some physical illnesses to grief or anger. Hippocrates believed that health depends upon a balance of the body, mind and environment, and that disease is caused by imbalances in these areas. As modern science progressed, the mind and emotions became neglected, since researchers found it difficult to measure and quantify mental states with the scientific methods and equipment that were so highly valued.

In the early 1900s, Harvard physiologist Walter Cannon coined the term "fight-or-flight response" for the body's reaction to threats, a response that causes increases in heart rate, blood pressure, blood sugar, muscle tension and respiration. During the 1950s, Hans Selye of McGill University pioneered research in what he called stress. Selye determined that the fight-or-flight response could be triggered by psychological factors as well as by physical threats. Stress includes having fight-or-flight reactions in situations where there is no immediate threat except mental perceptions and worries. Stress is not necessarily negative, except when people fail to cope with it effectively. Selye's work laid the groundwork for researchers to determine that stress and reactions to it play an integral role in health and disease.

Benefits

Mind/body therapies have shown promise in treating cancer, heart disease, hypertension, asthma, and mental illness. They have been used as effective complementary therapies alongside such conventional treatments as surgery and chemotherapy. Mind/body therapies have also been shown to increase quality of life, reduce pain, and improve symptoms for people with chronic diseases and health conditions. They may also help control and reverse certain diseases, particularly those that are stress-related. By reducing stress, mind/body therapies may even prevent many diseases. Another benefit of mind/body therapies is that they pose very little risk. Some are inexpensive, and most have few side effects.

There are many alternative techniques that draw upon the interconnections between mind and body. These include art therapy, assertiveness training, autogenic training, bioenergetics, biofeedback, breath therapy, mental imagery, dance and movement therapy, dreamwork, Gestalt therapy, group therapy, hypnosis, meditation, mindfulness training, Jungian psychoanalysis, postural integration, prayer and faith healing, progressive relaxation, psychodrama, psychotherapy, Reichian therapy, support groups, and yoga. Some of the most widely used techniques are meditation, mindfulness training, biofeedback, breath therapy, hypnosis, mental imagery, and movement therapies, which are discussed below.

Costs can vary widely for mind/body treatments, depending on the type and the medical training of the practitioner. Many insurance companies will reimburse some mind/body treatments and training sessions; consumers should be aware of their insurance provisions.

Biofeedback Therapy

Biofeedback is a self-regulation technique through which patients learn to voluntarily control what were once thought to be involuntary body processes. This intervention requires specialised equipment to convert physiological signals into meaningful visual and auditory cues, as well as a trained biofeedback practitioner to guide the therapy. Using a screen such as a computer monitor, patients get feedback that helps them develop control over their physiology. Just as looking into a mirror allows one to see and change positions, expressions, etc., biofeedback allows patients to see inside their bodies, with a trained practitioner serving as a guide directing them to use the feedback to regulate their physiology in a healthy direction.

Surface electromyography (sEMG) is perhaps the most common physiological variable monitored using biofeedback. sEMG feedback is used in a variety of disorders such as tension headache, chronic pain, spasmodic torticollis and temporomandibular joint dysfunction. Electroencephalography (EEG) feedback, also called neurofeedback, is used in ADHD and epilepsy and is increasingly the focus of research and other applications.

Some of the other commonly monitored variables are used when the goal of biofeedback is to reduce sympathetic arousal. These include heart rate, respiration rate, skin surface temperature (at the fingertips), skin conductance and heart rate variability. This physiological information is normally not viewed as being under conscious control, but biofeedback provides real-time data, helping to bring such physiological processes under the control of the patient. Common disorders treated in this way include hypertension, anxiety and medical conditions exacerbated by stress. Biofeedback also helps to make patients aware of the thoughts, feelings and behaviours related to their physiology. Over time, they can learn to self-regulate without feedback screens in front of them.

Two Models of Biofeedback Training

Biofeedback training is used in a variety of settings in order to improve academic, athletic and corporate performance, as well to improve health and wellness. This training may follow one of two learning models, each of which provides feedback so that the client learns techniques that help to correct any present malfunctioning.

Operant Conditioning and Feedback Learning

Operant conditioning is a model of learning which utilises consequences as a means to modify the occurrence or type of behavior. For biofeedback, a straight operant conditioning model relies solely on the reinforcement of the signal displays in order to prompt patients to change their physiology. Feedback learning often functions together with operant reinforcement. An example outside the healthcare arena is learning to putt a golf ball. As the individual sees where the ball goes, the feedback helps to improve the next stroke. In biofeedback, seeing the physiological data go in a better direction results in feedback learning, and positive reinforcement learning is usually satisfying. The therapist is simply there to explain what the biofeedback equipment is measuring and how it relates to the patient's physiology. Operant conditioning and the feedback learning model have been used in the management of many medical disorders including Raynaud's disease and faecal incontinence.

Psychophysiological Psychotherapy

Patients who are suffering from a disease that has a major stress component may also be helped by biofeedback using a psychophysiological psychotherapy model of learning. In this model, it is necessary to understand the patient as an individual. Stress management and other psychotherapeutic interventions may be used in combination with biofeedback training in order to make patients aware of how the stress in their lives has an effect on physiology. This model of learning uses both a psychophysiological assessment, described below, and a psychological evaluation in order to determine the thought and behaviour patterns that contribute to the patient's physiological vulnerability. This application of biofeedback training, which includes stress management, may be the most successful in treating stress related disorders.

Training Not Treatment

Biofeedback therapy is a process of training as opposed to a treatment. Much like being taught how to tie their shoes or ride a bicycle, individuals undergoing biofeedback training must take an active role and practise in order to develop the skill. Rather than passively receiving a treatment, the patient is an active learner. It's like learning a new language.

When a patient comes in for clinical biofeedback therapy, an emphasis is placed on education. As sensors are placed on the patient's skin, the therapist explains what each sensor will be measuring, assuring the patient that the sensors do not cause any pain or shock but rather are simply recording signals from the body and displaying those signals on the screen. The therapist chooses signal displays which take into account both the needs and limitations of the individual being seen, and then explains each signal. This may be as simple as 'the green line is muscle tension, the blue line is temperature', etc. Patients are then taught how the signals being displayed relate to their physiology. For example, the therapist may say, 'Raise your shoulders' or 'Scrunch your face,' using the muscle tension signal on the screen to point out the patient's physiological responses.

Patients are also shown how their physiology is reactive to mental stimuli, particularly stressful situations. This is often done with a psychophysiological assessment including a series of activities and recoveries. First patients are asked to relax, and then they are asked to engage in a stressful activity such as the Stroop Color–Word Test or the Serial Sevens Test before once again being asked to relax. The therapist can then pause the feedback and show the patient his or her physiological reactivity to the mental task, as well as the extent and speed with which the physiology returned to baseline values. At this point the therapist may explain what the optimal values are for each of the physiological variables being measured as well as how they relate to patient health. For example, the therapist may say, 'Keeping the green line down below two microvolts means that your muscles are already relaxed'. This may also be related to the patient's current condition by saying something such as 'If you practise letting go of the tension in these muscles, then you will experience headaches less frequently or with less intensity'. The therapist may then provide the patient with suggestions of how to use imagery or self-talk to reduce stress. The final aspect of biofeedback training is reinforcement by the therapist that the patient is doing a good job and is more in control of his or her recovery and wellness.

Indications for Referral

Individuals may be referred for biofeedback training as either an alternative or an adjunctive therapy. Current treatment may be producing an insufficient response or even no response at all. Individuals who are intolerant of medication or for whom pharmacological treatment is contraindicated (e.g. the patient is pregnant or may become pregnant, or the patient is breast feeding) may be referred for biofeedback training. Patients who for any reason are not adhering to their current treatment regimen may also respond to biofeedback training. Some patients may request additional help or therapy. Individuals who have stress as a significant component of their medical condition can be referred for biofeedback training combined with psychotherapy. There is also significant self-selection, as patients who value self-control are likely to ask for biofeedback or be most receptive when it is offered.

Biofeedback Gaining Popular Acceptance

Clinical biofeedback training is steadily gaining acceptance with the American public. Biofeedback is recognised by the National Institute of Complementary and Alternative Medicine as one of the mind–body therapies and many doctors and patients think of biofeedback as a form of complementary and alternative medicine (CAM). The last decade has demonstrated a significant increase in the prevalence of CAM use. A recent in-person survey of health-and illness-related experiences showed that in the USA alone, approximately 38% of adults and 12% of children are using some form of CAM for general healthcare and wellness or to treat a range of symptoms and diseases. In 2007, Americans spent nearly $34 billion on CAM practitioners and products.

As more and more Americans seek out such complementary and alternative therapies for their healthcare and as research continues to reveal the efficacy of biofeedback for more and more medical disorders, it is likely that it will become an accepted therapy for more disease conditions. A large study being undertaken this fall at the Cleveland Clinic, with funding from the Bakken Heart–Brain Institute, seeks to investigate the efficacy of biofeedback in treating three populations of patients – those with coronary artery disease, diabetes or multiple sclerosis. We hope to establish in these and other diseases that biofeedback is successful in improving quality of life and clinical status, as well as possibly reversing biological aspects of each disease.

Hypnosis

Although no consensus definition of hypnosis exists, the studies reviewed indicate that hypnosis involves the induction of a state of mind in which a person's normal critical or skeptical nature is bypassed, allowing for acceptance of suggestions. This state of heightened receptivity for suggestions (induction) is developed with the cooperation of the patient and is followed by the delivery of positive suggestions. Hypnosis is also described as an "attentive, receptive focal concentration," with the trance state being a "normal activity of a normal mind," which occurs regularly, as when reading an absorbing book, watching an engrossing movie, daydreaming, or performing monotonous activity. A common assumption is that, during hypnosis, the subconscious mind is in a suggestible state while the conscious mind is distracted or guided to become dormant.

Hypnosis may be compared with meditation, which generally is considered to involve a quieting of the mind. Meditation may be self-directed. If suggestions are given to achieve a desired effect, meditation may qualify as hypnosis depending on the state achieved, particularly because hypnosis can occur naturally (ie, without formal induction).

No attempt is made herein to explain the mechanism of hypnosis for causing the intended changes as a result of the suggestions given. If positive suggestions for change are accepted by the mind, any physiological changes that follow defy explanation by contemporary medicine, although complex explanations have been proposed.

Is Hypnosis Real?

Various methods have been used to determine whether hypnosis is a separate state, distinct from sleep, or if the patient is simply complying with the practitioner's instructions. Volunteers in whom hypnosis was induced were evaluated by positron emission tomography (PET). When subjects were given the suggestion to see color, the color perception areas of their cerebral hemispheres were activated whether they were looking at color or black-andwhite patterns. When subjects were given the suggestion to see black and white, the color perception areas of the brain showed decreased activity regardless of what the subjects were viewing. This implies that hypnosis is not a process of simply following instructions but actually involves a change in the brain's perception.

Characteristics of hypnosis and a hypnosis session.

Hypnosis is a state of mind that occurs naturally or is established by compliance with instructions and is characterized by:

- Focused attention.
- Heightened receptivity for suggestions.
- A bypass of the normal critical nature of the mind.
- Delivery of acceptable suggestions.

A hypnosis session consists of:

- An explanation of the process and consent.

- Induction of the trance state.
- Deepening of the trance.
- Assessment for adequacy of the trance.
- Hypnoanalysis—an investigative step (if necessary).
- Delivery of acceptable suggestions.
- Emergence from the trance state.

Studies have used other methods, such as electrodermal skin conductance, to evaluate whether patients in whom hypnosis was induced were "lying" or simply complying with instructions. Unpleasant sensations were noted on PET to cause activity in the anterior cingulate cortex. Hypnosis induced before painful stimuli caused a decrease in the subjective and objective perception of the pain as noted on the scans. Another study using PET in hypnotized persons showed activation of a region in the right anterior cingulate cortex (Brodmann area 32), an area activated when sound is heard or when sound is suggested in hypnosis but not when sound is simply imagined. This implies that the mind registered the hypnotic hallucination as if it were real. Other studies using PET support the occurrence of distinct changes in the brain with hypnosis. By using electroencephalography, changes were seen during hypnosis that could not be evoked by waking imagination.

Hypnosis does not act as a placebo (administering a pharmacologically inert substance). Studies using hypnosis for anesthesia indicate that pain relief from hypnosis is different from a placebo effect with evidence that the pain is not perceived rather than simply experienced with greater tolerance.

Hypnosis is not a state of sleep. Relaxation generally is believed to be a part of hypnosis, but it need not be. Volunteers underwent hypnotic induction with use of either the traditional method involving eye closure, relaxation, and drowsiness encouraged by suggestion or an active, alert method involving riding a stationary bicycle while receiving suggestions for alertness and activity. Equally receptive trance states were achieved by the relaxation and alert methods, and examples were presented of other active, alert trance states. Of note, hypnotized patients may experience considerable anxiety and other emotions while reliving an event with age regression without coming out of the trance state.

Age regression, inducing a person through hypnosis to relive events that occurred earlier in life, is believed to differ from enhancement of memory, but scientific evidence for this assertion is limited. Age regression may be helpful to treat conditions in which an adverse behavior is believed to be based on a past event; however, its validity is controversial. The process of regression may generate strong emotions and can possibly alter a memory or create a false memory. Studies about the use of age regression have reported the development of infantile neurologic reflexes on regression to infancy, agespecific handwriting and vocabularies on regression to childhood, and knowledge of the appropriate day of the week of events in the period to which the person was regressed.

Modern Hypnosis

The era of modern hypnotism began with the Austrian physician Franz Anton Mesmer, who is said to have brought animal magnetism (the term for hypnosis at that time) to France in 1778. Because many people were seeking treatment from Mesmer and his colleagues, King Louis XVI of France commissioned Benjamin Franklin and others to investigate the practice. After extensive testing, the commission discredited Mesmer, indicating in their report that any medical benefit was not from magnetism, as publicized, and that mesmerism involved only "imagination, imitation, and touch." One account indicates that Thomas Jefferson obtained copies of the report to help prevent the spread of mesmerism to America.

This setback for hypnosis led to a deeper, more covert evaluation of the process. James Braid, using eye fixation techniques, was able to produce a trance state and later discovered the importance of adding suggestions. He is credited with introducing the term hypnotism, although he favored monoideism because he realized that the state differs from sleep. In the 19th century, the English surgeon John Elliotson and the Scottish surgeon James Esdaile performed hundreds of surgical procedures with use of hypnosis for anesthesia and with extremely low morbidity rates for the times. Almost simultaneously with the reports of success with hypnosis, ether and chloroform became popular and displaced the use of hypnosis for anesthesia in surgery. Twentieth-century hypnosis was influenced by the contrasting techniques of indirect suggestion intermixed with psychoanalysis promoted by Milton H. Erickson and of direct suggestion and induction of a deep trance state for age regression espoused by others.

Acceptance of Hypnosis in Medicine

Acceptance of hypnosis in medicine has evolved slowly. In 1847, the Roman Catholic Church indicated acceptance of hypnosis, noting that hypnosis was not morally forbidden, and in 1956, Pope Pius XII noted its use for childbirth and indicated the need for proper precautions as for other forms of medical treatment. Other religions (with exceptions) have shown acceptance, with ministers of different faiths trained in and using hypnosis in their practices.

In 1958, the American Medical Association (AMA) published and approved a report from a 2-year study by the Council on Mental Health. The report indicated that there can be "definite and proper uses of hypnosis in medical and dental practice" and recommended the establishment of "necessary training facilities" in the United States. The British Medical Association had issued its report on hypnosis in the

British Medical Journal in 1955, with which the AMA's Council on Mental Health indicated "essential agreement." The American Psychiatric Association, in a position statement approved by the Council of the Association in 1961, indicated that "hypnosis has definite application in the various fields of medicine" and that physicians would be seeking psychiatrists for training in hypnosis. A National Institutes of Health panel issued a statement published by the AMA in 1996 indicating that there was "strong evidence for the use of hypnosis in alleviating pain associated with cancer."

Risks of Hypnosis

A few cases of patients who displayed "unanticipated" adverse behavior after hypnosis. Adverse reactions or hypnotic complications consisted of "unexpected, unwanted thoughts, feelings or behaviors during or after hypnosis which are inconsistent with agreed goals and interfere with the hypnotic process by impairing optimal mental function." The most common suspected adverse reactions included drowsiness, dizziness, stiffness, headaches, anxiety, and, occasionally, more serious reactions such as symptom substitution and masking of organic disorders. These adverse reactions were attributed to deficiencies in the hypnotist's techniques, such as not realizing that suggestions in hypnosis are accepted literally, bringing the patient too rapidly out of trance, using age regression inappropriately, not dispelling preconceived expectations of negative consequences of hypnosis before initiating the session, or not prescreening for certain psychopathology. A more recent review indicated that hypnosis is associated with a risk of adverse effects, including headache, dizziness, nausea, anxiety, or panic, at levels that might occur in other test or experimental settings without hypnosis. A prehypnosis discussion session with the patient was advocated. It has been argued that informed consent is not needed before casual or brief techniques involving helpful semantics since the use of careless and harmful comments from health care workers has no such prerequisite. Hypnosis generally is considered a "benign process" with "few contraindications"; however, pseudomemories can be created if leading questions are asked during the investigative phase of hypnosis.

Evaluation of the Clinical Trials

Evaluation of clinical trials of hypnosis is complicated by the nature of hypnosis. The gold standard of a randomized, double-blind, controlled trial is virtually impossible because cooperation and rapport between patient and therapist are needed to achieve a receptive trance state. The few hypnosis trials that were blinded involved suggestions delivered by audiotape during surgery while patients were under general anesthesia (assumed to be a hypnoticlike state). Evaluation of these trials is limited by the lack of standardized techniques for hypnotic induction, evaluation of the level of trance, delivery of suggestions, or number and length of sessions. Although the state of hypnosis involves increased receptivity to acceptable suggestions, the methods of delivering the suggestions vary substantially. In some trials, researchers gave suggestions only for relaxation or no suggestions at all. In other trials, researchers indirectly suggested that patients allow a feeling or imagination rather than directing them to have a certain feeling, which relied on patients understanding the intention. In some studies, researchers gave suggestions only to distract the mind during an otherwise uncomfortable procedure or condition.

Thus, it is reasonable to consider the appropriateness of judging hypnosis by the best or worst results, with use of averaging, or by meta-analyses. Indeed, although better methods would be expected to achieve better results, many trials gave too few details about technique to allow comparison. If the most efficacious hypnosis techniques were known, a more representative review of the state of the art may include only trials using such techniques.

A deficiency of the trials reviewed is the lack of randomization of patient and practitioner variables that may affect outcome. Patient characteristics such as fear, attentiveness, interest, expectation, suggestibility, motivation, desire, and belief in hypnosis may alter outcomes. According to the literature, vital practitioner characteristics in clude training and experience and the ability to induce trance, to properly word suggestions, and to establish the necessary states of expectancy, rapport, and motivation (if not already present). Furthermore, results from clinical trials may not accurately estimate the effectiveness achievable in an office setting with willing, expectant patients. In clinical trials, many patients are likely to be unwilling, unmotivated, or skeptical about hypnosis. Hypnosis appears to be "particularly useful and yields better results when it is specifically requested by the patient." Consequently, clinical trials may underestimate the benefits of hypnosis compared with those obtainable by a proficient, experienced hypnotist.

Clinical Trials of Hypnosis

Allergy

Allergic or hypersensitivity reactions usually are not believed to be psychosomatic and thus are generally considered as unable to be influenced by suggestion. These highly complex reactions involve IgE antibodies, activation of mast cells and basophils, and release of chemical mediators of inflammatory and immune responses. Some early literature suggested that many allergies might have an emotional basis and thus be treatable by hypnosis. Subsequent studies have shown that hypnosis may alter the body's physiological response to various stimuli. In a study of 18 volunteers selected for their hypnotizability, immediate-type hypersensitivity reactions were suppressed in 8 of the 12 patients given brief direct suggestions in hypnosis. In another trial, hypnotic suggestions for relaxation reduced helper/inducer cell percentages, helper/suppressor cell ratios, and natural killer cell activity compared with prehypnosis baseline values. Other researchers have shown the positive effects of social support on natural killer cell activity and cortisol levels and the adverse effects of stress in patients with cancer, which has implications for cancer progression.

Skin prick testing for type I (immediate) hypersensitivity and testing with purified protein derivative (in persons vaccinated previously for tuberculosis) for type IV hypersensitivity were performed before and after hypnosis.39 Patients in the hypnosis group (but not the control group) who were given suggestions for increasing or decreasing skin reactions were able to increase the flare and wheal reactions on 1 arm and decrease the flare reaction on the other, with a significant difference between the 2 arms. The same authors later studied volunteers selected for their high hypnotizability and evaluated their reactions to histamine pin pricks and laser-induced burn pain. Hypnosis was associated with a significant reduction in both pain and flare reactions.

Anesthesia for Pain Relief

Numerous studies have shown benefits of hypnosis for pain relief. In a study with experimental pain stimulation by pin prick and laser heat, direct suggestions in hypnosis resulted in a significant decrease in pain, measured subjectively and objectively by means of pain-related brain potentials. In another study, highly hypnotizable (based on susceptibility testing) volunteers given painful electrical stimulation were able to increase or decrease their perception of pain as noted on event-related somatosensory potentials.

The mechanism of analgesia from hypnosis appears to differ significantly from a placebo effect and from induced endorphin production (endogenous opiates). The morphine antagonist naloxone does not block the pain relief afforded by hypnosis. In a small study, pain was produced in highly hypnotizable volunteers by inflating a blood pressure cuff on the upper arm to 250 mm Hg followed by exercise and leaving the cuff on for 10 minutes. All patients reported a pain level of 8 or more (on a scale of 0 to 10, with 10 being the most intense) before hypnosis. With hypnosis, all reported a pain level of 0, and this relief was not altered substantially by administration of naloxone.

Hypnosis for pain relief in the clinical setting appears to have similar benefit. In a randomized, double-blind (for the use of naloxone) crossover study, patients with neuropathic pain were taught self-hypnosis. Considerable relief from pain was achieved by hypnosis, and this relief was not reversed by administration of naloxone. In patients with low hypnotizability, hypnosis was equal to placebo for pain relief, whereas highly hypnotizable people benefited more from hypnosis than from placebo. This finding indicates that hypnosis involves at least 2 effects: a placebo-type effect and one in which suggestion distorts perception.

Pain relief afforded by hypnosis differs from that induced by acupuncture. Twenty volunteers were evaluated for the level of pain caused by 2 different experimentally induced methods and were treated subsequently with hypnosis, acupuncture, medication, or placebo. Hypnosis with direct suggestions for pain relief produced significant pain relief compared with placebo ($P < 0.001$) and gave the best results of all the treatments. The most favorable results with hypnosis tended to be in those who were highly hypnotizable, whereas the results with acupuncture were not related to hypnotizability. Patients with head and neck pain studied in a single crossover trial served as their own controls before and after treatment with hypnosis or acupuncture. Both treatments were effective in relieving pain, although patients believed to have psychogenic pain fared better with hypnosis, and those who were apprehensive about hypnosis had less benefit.

Table: Comparison of clinical trials of hypnosis for analgesia.

Type of pain	Testing for hypno-tiz-ability	Trial		No. of subjects/ patients	Refractory condition	Self hypnosis or home tapes?	Therapy	No. of sessions	Follow up
		Controlled	Randomized						
Induced by tourniquet	Yes	Own†	No	3	NA	No	Individual	1	NA
Neuropathic	Yes	Own†	Double-blind, cross over	6	No	Yes	NR	NR	NA
Induced by ice water or tourniquet	Yes	Own†	No	20	NA	No	Individual	1	NA
Various: head and neck	Yes	Own†	Cross over	25	Some	Yes	Individual then audiotapes	3	None
Burn wounds	No	Yes	Yes	42	No	Yes	Individual then self hypnosis	Variable	NR
Burn wounds	No	Yes	Yes	57	No	No	Individual	1	None
Temporo-mandibular disorders	No	Own†	Yes	23	Yes	Yes	Group	6	6 mo

*NA = not applicable; NR = not reported.

†Patients served as their own controls.

‡Patients encouraged to use either self-hypnosis or audiotapes at home (usually daily).

Many trials have evaluated hypnosis for pain relief for burn injuries. A review of the use of hypnosis for severely burned children encouraged its use for pain and prevention of regressive behavior and included case reports. Clinical trials have shown significant pain relief with hypnosis in patients with burns, many of whom were taught self-hypnosis for pain control. In one trial, patients were treated with a single session of hypnosis. Those with severe pain (but not those with less pain) noted significant pain relief compared with controls. As in some other studies, younger patients tended to have better results. Adult patients with recalcitrant temporomandibular joint pain treated with hypnosis with suggestions for jaw relaxation noted significant pain reduction, which persisted at the 6- month follow-up.

A meta-analysis published in 2000 evaluated the use of hypnosis for pain relief in the preceding 20 years. That review of 18 studies indicated that hypnosis offered a moderate to large analgesic effect for many types of pain, which met "the criteria for well established treatment." Because hypnosis was noted to benefit most patients, a broader application of its use was advocated. A 2003 comprehensive review of hypnosis for pain relief found it superior to placebo for acute pain and at times superior to pain relief achieved by other means. Hypnosis for chronic pain was concluded to be a viable option, with the understanding that pain therapy requires "multidimensional assessment and treatment."

Anesthesia for Surgery

Hypnosis has been used as the sole agent of anesthesia for both major and minor surgical procedures. In the 19th century, John Elliotson and James Esdaile reported their successful use of mesmerism for anesthesia in hundreds of operations, with decreased mortality compared with other methods. Nonetheless, they were censored by the medical community at the time for unacceptable techniques. Instead, chloroform, nitrous oxide, and ether won acceptance for general anesthesia.

The use of hypnosis as the sole agent for anesthesia has been virtually abandoned because of the availability and dependability of pharmacological agents; nevertheless, a few such cases have been described in contemporary medical literature. Hypnoanalgesia was described for repair of atrial septal defects in 3 patients and for mitral commissurotomy in 4 patients, with hypnosis as the sole method of anesthesia for 1 of the patients. The patients were able to open and close their eyes on command during surgery and to extubate themselves postoperatively. An oral surgeon documented his own cholecystectomy performed with use of only self-hypnosis for anesthesia. He walked back to his room after surgery and returned to work on the 10th postoperative day.

Table: Comparison of clinical trials of hypnosis for anesthesia.

Testing for hypnotizability*	No. of patients	Self-hypnosis†
No	60	No
No	20	No
No	241	Yes
No	30	Yes
Yes	32	No

*In all these randomized, controlled trials, hypnosis treatment consisted of 1 individual therapy session, and there was no follow-up.

†Patients encouraged to use self-hypnosis during the procedure.

A 1999 review of more than 1650 surgical cases using hypnosis combined with other methods for conscious sedation promoted the safety and patient comfort afforded by hypnosis. This form of anesthesia was used instead of general anesthesia for a broad range of surgical procedures, including thyroidectomy, cervicotomy for hyperparathyroidism, breast augmentation, neck lift, correction of mammary ptosis, nasal septorhinoplasty, débridement with skin grafting, maxillofacial reconstruction, and tubal ligation. The authors concluded that hypnosis prevents pharmacological unconsciousness, allows patient participation, and may allow a faster recovery and a shorter hospital stay but requires some changes in the atmosphere of the operating room because of the conscious state of the patient. Other studies support the multiple benefits of hypnosis as an adjunct to conscious sedation for many types of surgery.

Brief hypnosis has been documented to be beneficial for anesthesia before excisional breast biopsies and invasive radiological procedures. Similar benefit was afforded to patients taught self-hypnosis, which was used during radiological procedures. In a randomized trial, patients hypnotized before and during coronary artery angioplasty required less pain medication and had a mild increase in tolerance to balloon-induced ischemia. Benefit was observed, presumably from the relaxed state and from distraction, without specific suggestions given for not feeling discomfort.

Dermatology

Many trials have evaluated hypnosis for eliminating warts; however, evaluation is complicated by spontaneous remission rates of 20% to 45% and by accounts of warts being produced by suggestion. Fourteen patients with bilateral warts for at least 6 months were given direct suggestions for only unilateral clearing of the warts. Of the 10 patients who were able to reach at least a moderate depth of hypnosis, (64% of the total group) achieved complete or near-complete resolution of the warts at 3-month follow-up. The warts on the contralateral side were not affected except in 1 highly hypnotizable person whose contralateral warts resolved 6 weeks later. Hypnosis was advocated to avoid pain and scarring, reactions to anesthetics, and the need for wound care and special equipment. The technique may be particularly applicable for warts in sensitive or inaccessible areas.

In a case report of 41 consecutive patients with predominantly refractory warts, direct suggestions in hypnosis, followed by age-regression techniques for any nonresponders, resulted in a cure rate of 80% with no recurrences. In volunteers with warts on the hand, a significant difference was seen in the rate of remission in those treated with hypnosis (50%) compared with that in the control group (12%). Hypnotizability was not found to be related to successful remission, whereas low expectation for wart regression had a negative association. Volunteers assigned to receive hypnosis had significantly fewer warts at the 6- week follow-up evaluation than did groups treated with either placebo or salicylic acid.

Hypnosis has been used successfully for other dermatologic conditions. Patients with atopic dermatitis noted decreased pruritus, scratching, sleep disturbance, and tension after treatment with hypnosis. In many patients, improvements persisted at follow-up evaluations up to 18 months later. A review of the use of hypnosis in dermatology supports its value for many skin conditions not believed to be under conscious control.

Gastroenterology

Hypnosis for irritable bowel syndrome (IBS) has been studied extensively. A 1984 study in England showed significant benefits from hypnosis. Thirty patients with refractory IBS and severe symptoms were randomly assigned to 7 individual sessions of hypnotherapy or psychotherapy plus placebo pills. Although the psychotherapy group showed a small but significant improvement in some characteristics, all patients in the hypnosis group had significant improvements ($P < 0.001$) in well-being, bowel habits, distention symptoms, and pain, with no relapses at 3-month follow-up. A subsequent report added 35 more patients to the hypnosis group of 15 from the earlier study; those with classic symptoms and no psychological problems fared best with hypnosis, as did patients younger than 50 years. Direct, specific suggestions for symptom relief were most successful. At 18-month followup, the 15 patients in the earlier hypnosis group remained in remission.

Table: Comparison of clinical trials of hypnosis for warts.

Testing for hypnotizability	Trial		No. of patients	Refractory condition	Self-hypnosis or home tapes†	No. of sessions	Follow up
	Controlled	Randomized					
Yes	Own‡	No	14	Some	No	Not reported	3 mo
No	No	No	41	Most	No	Variable	6 mo to several years
Yes	Yes	Yes	63	No	No	1 individual, 1 self	6 wk
Yes	Yes	Yes	40	No	No	1 individual plus self	6 wk

*In each trial, individual therapy was used.

†Patients encouraged to use either self-hypnosis or audiotapes at home (usually daily).

‡The contralateral side was the control.

The positive results with hypnosis for IBS have been confirmed in several other trials. It was concluded that "in addition to relieving the symptoms of irritable bowel syndrome, hypnotherapy profoundly improves the patients' quality of life and reduces absenteeism from work." Use of audiotapes for self-hypnosis at home, used in many IBS studies, was considered important for success. Other studies and reviews have shown similar results for IBS.

Patients with peptic ulcer disease have benefited from hypnosis. Thirty patients with recurrent peptic ulcer disease were treated with ranitidine and were assigned randomly to receive hypnosis or ranitidine alone, initiated after healing was documented by esophagogastroduodenoscopy. During 12 months of monitoring, significantly fewer patients in the hypnosis group (53%) experienced relapse compared with 100% of patients in the ranitidine-only group. The benefit may be from suppression of the secretion of gastric acid, as shown by a study of 32 volunteers who were able to significantly and appropriately increase and decrease gastric acid secretion (compared with their baseline values) from suggestive imagery in hypnosis. In a study of 126 patients with functional dyspepsia, those treated with hypnosis noted improvement in quality of life and long-term symptoms, fewer physician visits, and less health care spending compared with the group treated with medication.

Postoperative gastrointestinal motility has been affected positively by hypnosis. Patients scheduled to undergo abdominal surgery were assigned randomly to either a treat ment group read suggestions for an early return of bowel function and appetite or a control group given only general preoperative instructions for an equal period. With their surgeons unaware of the study, patients who were read a 5- minute script before surgery had a significantly earlier return of bowel function ($P < .05$) They also had a shorter mean duration of hospital stay (6.6 vs 8.1 days) and a cost savings of $1200 per patient. Patients in the perioperative state, as well as patients treated in the emergency department, are alleged to be in a highly receptive or hypnoticlike state not requiring formal hypnotic induction. The use of positive assertions during a situation in which the patient is reliant on and receptive to the health care practitioner, but not in a formal trance state, has been termed waking hypnosis.

Testing for hypnotiz-ability	Trial		No. of patients	Refrac-tory con-dition	Self-hyp-nosis or home tapes*	Therapy	No. of sessions	Follow up
	Con-trolled	Ran-dom-ized						
No	Yes	Yes	30	Yes	Yes	Individual	7	3 mo
No	No	No	35	Yes	Yes	Individual	≤10	≤18 mo
No	No	Yes	33	Yes	Yes	Group vs individual	4	5 mo
No	Yes	No	30	No	No	Individual	10	3 mo
No	Yes	No	50	Yes	Yes	Individual	12	Not reported

Yes	Yes	Yes	12	Some	Yes	Individual	12	Not reported
No	Own†	No	27	Yes	Yes	Individual	12	Variable
No	Own†	No	250	Yes	Yes	Individual	12	3 mo

*Patients encouraged to use either self-hypnosis or audiotapes at home (usually daily).

†Patients served as their own controls.

Hypnosis has been used alone or in combination as anesthesia for liver biopsy, esophagogastroduodenoscopy, and colonoscopy. A gastroenterologist reported the use of only an anesthetic throat spray and hypnosis for 200 upper gastrointestinal tract endoscopy procedures with a reduced overall duration of the procedure. No complications were noted, and patients were able to leave immediately afterward. In another report, patients with either anxiety or allergy to local anesthetics safely underwent liver biopsies with use of hypnosis. Half the patients in a pilot trial reached a moderate or deep level of hypnosis before colonoscopic evaluations, with more than 80% noting only mild or no discomfort.

Healing from Surgery or Injury

Two trials evaluated the potential for hypnotic suggestions to facilitate faster wound healing after injuries or surgery. A pilot trial of hypnosis for patients with nondisplaced ankle fractures showed marginally faster healing, diminished pain, and increased mobility and functionality. Eighteen presurgical patients were assigned randomly to a hypnosis group that received positive suggestions for healing, a control group that received supportive attention to the patients' concerns, or a standard care group. Surgeons were unaware of their treatment group. Patients in the hypnosis group showed significantly improved healing at 1 and 7 weeks postoperatively compared with the other groups ($P<.02$).

Hematology

One medical center reported favorable results with the addition of hypnosis for patients with hemophilia. Patients who were assigned to receive hypnosis had a significantly decreased need for transfusions compared with controls ($P =.01$). A review of this program described the methods and various benefits of teaching self-hypnosis to these patients.

Hypertension

Few studies have evaluated the use of hypnosis for hypertension. In 1 study of 44 patients, the hypnosis group had a significant decrease in blood pressure compared with the control group. At 6 months, the hypnosis group had mean decreases of 13.3 mm Hg systolic and 8.5 mm Hg diastolic below their baseline blood pressures.

Neurology

Hypnosis has been used successfully for treatment of headaches. Patients with chronic (≥6 months) tension headaches were assigned randomly to hypnosis or a control group. The hypnosis group had a significant reduction in the number, duration, and intensity of headaches. Instruction in self-hypnosis produced significant benefit for tension headaches in other studies including a group of less hypnotizable patients. Hypnosis was compared with propranolol use for children with migraine headaches in a prospective, randomized, controlled, crossover trial. Patients taught self-hypnosis had a decreased frequency of headaches. In another trial, university students with chronic headaches were studied. Hypnosis using imagery for relaxation and serenity was compared with an active placebo that consisted of watching slides falsely claimed to contain potent subliminal messages for pain relief. Both groups achieved significant ($P < .05$) and equal decreases in headache pain compared with controls. Hypnosis did not outperform the placebo; however, the hypnosis group received no specific suggestions for pain relief, whereas the placebo group was given suggestions to expect such benefit (waking hypnosis).

Obesity

Studies of hypnosis as a single treatment for obesity show variable and limited success. A critical review of hypnosis for obesity in studies from 1958 through 1978 concluded that hypnosis may be of benefit but that standardization of methods was needed. In a subsequent trial with 156 participants, results from participants who received 9 weekly individual hypnosis sessions plus behavior-modification treatments were compared with results from those who received behavior-modification treatment alone. On average, the hypnosis group had lost 7 kg of weight more than the control group at the 2-year follow-up. A meta-analysis of trials in the 1980s showed significantly greater weight loss for those treated with hypnosis and behavior therapy compared with those who received behavior therapy alone, and this effect persisted or increased with time ($P < .05$) In another trial, 60 obese patients with sleep apnea were assigned randomly to treatment with diet alone or diet and hypnosis.98 Patients assigned to hypnosis (two 30-minute hypnosis sessions and a home audiotape) achieved signifi cant weight loss at 18 months ($P < .02$) however, the sleep apnea was not eliminated. Rather than a sole treatment for obesity, hypnosis may be more helpful as part of a program that includes arousing motivation, dietary counseling, and peer support.

Obstetrics

Hypnosis as anesthesia for childbirth has a long, successful history supported by several trials. A large trial compared a self-hypnosis group with a control group to study the effects of hypnosis on labor. The hypnosis group reported less discomfort and shortened labor. The women's volunteer status and the skill of the hypnotist were factors deemed important for success. Pregnant adolescents were assigned randomly to individual sessions of hypnosis or to supportive counseling with the medical staff blinded to their group assignments. At delivery, the hypnosis group had a significant decrease in complications, fewer surgical interventions, and a shorter hospital stay. Additional positive findings not statistically significant were a decreased need for anesthesia, postpartum analgesia, and infant admissions to the intensive care unit. In another trial, the use of a single session of hypnosis (and encouraging home use of an audiotape) did not induce delivery in postterm women. Patients with hyperemesis gravidarum have benefited from hypnotic intervention, according to 2 reviews with case reports.

Oncology

Chemotherapy often is associated with nausea and vomiting. Hypnosis has been studied for reducing these and other adverse effects. Children receiving chemotherapy who were assigned randomly to hypnosis had less anticipatory nausea and vomiting and less vomiting with chemotherapy compared with a control group. A later prospective randomized trial examined the effects of hypnosis for the adverse effects of chemotherapy in children with a resultant significant decrease in anticipatory nausea and the need for antiemetic medications. Children who learned self-hypnosis techniques were believed to have gained feelings of control over their situations.

Hypnosis has been used successfully in other areas of oncology. Patients undergoing bone marrow transplantation treated with hypnosis experienced significantly less oral pain than control patients.106 Patients with metastatic breast cancer benefited from self-hypnosis and from participation in group support. Despite a lack of specific suggestions, the women benefited with significantly less pain and an increased duration of survival. An untapped potential for hypnosis for cancer treatment is the reported ability to alter regional blood flow, which offers the prospect of increasing the delivery of chemotherapy to a tumor or reducing blood flow to it.

Otorhinolaryngology

Patients with chronic tinnitus treated with hypnosis improved significantly in 7 of 10 disturbing symptoms compared with a group treated with masking techniques or supportive measures ($P < 0.05$) These results support the findings from other trials.

Pulmonary Medicine

Several trials have evaluated hypnosis for asthma. A study of 55 patients with asthma noted that patients assigned randomly to the hypnosis group used bronchodilators less frequently and experienced less wheezing than controls. Those responding best were younger, more compliant with practicing self-hypnosis techniques, and more easily hypnotized, and they developed a deeper level of trance. Males responded as well as females, a finding not consistent in hypnosis trials. A large multicenter trial of patients with asthma reported a significant decrease in the number of treatment failures and a larger number of patients deemed "much improved" by independent assessment in the group taught self-hypnosis. Females in the hypnosis group also had lower wheezing scores and less use of bronchodilators. A retrospective study of asthmatic patients reported similar benefit, with 54% of patients treated with hypnosis having an "excellent" result and 21% becoming symptom free and discontinuing medication.

Decreased rates of hospital admissions, length of stay, and use of corticosteroids were attained with hypnotherapy during the year of study in patients with refractory asthma who served as their own controls. Highly hypnotizable patients assigned randomly to hypnosis for asthma treatment improved significantly in measurements of pulmonary function and noted improved symptoms and less use of bronchodilators compared with a control group.

A few cases have been reported of success with hypnosis in weaning dependent patients from ventilators. The report indicates a potential benefit of hypnosis when other techniques have failed.

Numerous studies have reported various techniques and outcomes in the use of hypnosis for smoking cessation, many with beneficial results. A 1970 study used a single 12-hour group session for volunteer smokers who had unsuccessfully tried other methods of smoking cessation. The program achieved an 88% 1-year abstention rate. In a large trial involving 615 persons unable to quit smoking published the same year, participants were taught self-hypnosis in a single, individual, 45-minute session. A 20% abstention rate was noted by questionnaire at 6 months, counting nonresponders as failures (45% abstention rate in the responders). Further studies patterned after this trial showed 31% to 40% abstention rates at 6 months.

In a 1992 meta-analysis of 633 smoking-cessation studies involving almost 72,000 participants, hypnosis was the most successful cessation method, with a 12% to 60% success rate (mean, 36%), 3.5 times that achieved by selfcare methods. More aggressive but less acceptable techniques that combined hypnosis with aversion methods (rapid smoking with negative imagery and electrical shocks) for smoking cessation resulted in a 3-month abstention rate of 86% in male volunteers and 87% in female volunteers. Another study that combined hypnosis with aversion methods reported a 90% abstention rate (39 of 43 consecutive referral patients) at 6 to 36 months.

Two studies examined the effect of suggestions for smoking cessation delivered during elective surgery. In a double-blind trial, patients listened to audiotapes during general anesthesia containing either simple, direct suggestions to stop smoking or simple counting without suggestions. After 1 month, significantly more patients in the suggestion group (8 patients) had stopped smoking compared with no patients in the control group (P < .005) No patient could actively recall the message on the tape. This study is one of several supporting the assertion that postoperative behavior can be influenced by suggestions given during general anesthesia without conscious recall of the suggestions. In contrast, another trial using a longer, complex message showed no difference in the smoking cessation rate between the treatment and control groups postoperatively.

Rheumatology

Patients with refractory fibromyalgia (mean duration, 8.5 years) who were randomly assigned to receive hypnosis obtained significant improvement compared with those assigned randomly to physical therapy alone. Benefits included improvements in morning fatigue (P =.003), sleep (P <.001) muscle pain (P =.004), overall assessment (P =.04), and use of pain medications, with results persisting for at least 6 months.

Surgery

A report from the 1960s indicated that surgical patients should be considered in a state of hypnosis and suggested that patients were able to comprehend much of the conversation around them, even while under anesthesia. In the perioperative state, the patient is fixated on the forthcoming process and is in a receptive, compliant state of mind, comparable to the state formally induced with hypnosis. The report further cautioned that patients in this receptive state may interpret comments made within an audible range as having negative implications for them if these comments are not made correctly. More recently, it has been emphasized again that health care personnel should be aware that patients under anesthesia have unconscious auditory perception and tend to interpret comments negatively. The report also stressed that, along with the potential deleterious effects of this awareness, came the opportunity for using "semantics of positive suggestion" (emphasizing comfort, safety, and success) that should be "an integral part" of surgical and obstetrical care. It appears appropriate to consider the use of suggestions for patients in the perioperative period as a part of the practice of hypnosis.

The subject of awareness under anesthesia is controversial. Much of the medical literature asserts that awareness under general anesthesia occurs only in rare cases, is indicative of an inadequate level of anesthesia, and can cause psychological trauma, presumably from fear induced during the awareness. A prospective study examined the possibility of patient awareness of events or comments occurring during anesthesia that may not be recalled consciously. Patients undergoing coronary artery bypass grafting surgery were assigned randomly to listen to either a personalized audiotape with specific instructions to be recalled postoperatively or no tape (control) during surgery. Postoperative hypnosis demonstrated significant (P=.01 compared with the control group) recall of material from the audiotape (as well as events during surgery) that was not recalled consciously. Numerous studies support the contention that patients have awareness under anesthesia that can affect their postoperative course.

Because it may be harmful to make comments within the audible range of surgical patients that may be perceived negatively by the patient, promoting good health by making comments of a clearly positive nature appears warranted. The "opportunity for positive semantics" was investigated in a randomized, double-blind study in which patients undergoing hysterectomy listened either to an audiotape with positive suggestions or to a blank tape while under general anesthesia. The treatment group had significantly fewer bowel problems ($P<.03$), shorter recovery time ($P<.002$), shorter hospital stay ($P<.002$), less fever ($P<.005$), and a better recovery (by nursing assessment) ($P<.002$) than the control patients. Other studies cited in the report indicated not only that "inappropriate or misinterpreted operating theatre comments may have a harmful effect upon recovery," but also that this perioperative awareness "may instead be employed to the benefit of the patient." Compared with matched controls, patients listening to positive suggestions before and during surgery had less blood loss and a shorter recovery. Recommendations for positive semantics for preoperative patients are similar to those applicable to emergency department patients. Persons in both situations appear to be in a hypnotic-like state (receptive, focused, willing to comply) and thus are particularly susceptible to remarks by health care workers.

Preoperative hypnosis is less controversial than the idea of awareness during anesthesia, with benefit noted in many trials. Significant benefits include less anxiety and decreased blood pressure reduced blood loss, enhanced postoperative well-being, improved intestinal motility, shorter hospital stay, reduced postoperative nausea and vomiting, and reduced need for analgesics. Substantial but not statistically significant decreases in cost and length of hospital stay were observed in another study.

A 1991 review of clinical trials using hypnosis, suggestion, or relaxation in the care of surgical patients found that 89% of the trials showed that these techniques produced a positive outcome in facilitating physical or psychological recovery from surgery. The use of live therapists (rather than suggestions from audiotapes) and positive and appropriate semantics (avoiding words that bring to mind undesired outcomes) at the most receptive times were advocated to foster shorter hospital stays, earlier recovery, and improved patient well-being. A meta-analysis published in 2002 evaluated hypnosis for surgical patients for its overall effect and benefits for specific clinical outcomes. Hypnosis as an adjunct to surgery was believed to be "successful for the majority of individuals," with benefits such as decreased pain, anxiety, nausea, and recovery time.

Urology

The medical literature from the 1960s indicated a strong potential for the use of hypnosis for impotence, and support for this assertion has come from recent clinical trials. A review of the personal experience and techniques of an experienced practitioner cited an 88% success rate using hypnosis for impotence in almost 3000 patients. The hypnosis techniques used in this trial were studied in 2 randomized controlled trials of men with nonorganic impotence. One trial that compared hypnosis with placebo showed an

80% improvement in sexual function with hypnosis compared with 36% with placebo. The second trial compared hypnosis with acupuncture and injected or oral placebo. The success rate (moderate improvement or "cure") was 75% for hypnosis. A review of developments in hypnosis reported its efficacy in augmenting other treatment methods for sexual dysfunction and its potential for exploring contributing psychological conflicts.

In a trial of hypnosis for chronic (mean, 7 years) urinary incontinence, 50 women served as their own controls. At 1 month, 58% were symptom-free and another 28% were improved, with cystometric testing at 3 months objectively confirming the benefits.

The acceptance of hypnosis as a mode of treatment in medicine is increasing as a result of "careful, methodical, empirical work of many research pioneers." Many important trials reviewed here have helped to establish the role of hypnosis in contemporary medicine. These trials have established the utility and efficacy of hypnosis for several medical conditions, either alone or as part of the treatment regimen. Nonetheless, skepticism may prevail and hypnosis may remain underused because of the tendency to doubt or fear the unknown. According to a recent study, health care providers changed their attitudes significantly and positively when presented with information about the use of hypnosis in medicine. Through greater awareness and acceptance of hypnosis, additional training and research can be inspired in pursuit of improved techniques and new areas of potential benefit.

Meditation

Meditation is a mind and body practice that has a long history of use for increasing calmness and physical relaxation, improving psychological balance, coping with illness, and enhancing overall health and well-being. Mind and body practices focus on the interactions among the brain, mind, body, and behavior. A new report based on data from the 2017 National Health Interview Survey (NHIS) found that U.S. adults' use of meditation in the past 12 months tripled between 2012 and 2017 (from 4.1 percent to 14.2 percent). The use of meditation by U.S. children (aged 4 to 17 years) also increased significantly (from 0.6 percent in 2012 to 5.4 percent in 2017).

There are many types of meditation, but most have four elements in common: a quiet location with as few distractions as possible; a specific, comfortable posture (sitting, lying down, walking, or in other positions); a focus of attention (a specially chosen word or set of words, an object, or the sensations of the breath); and an open attitude (letting distractions come and go naturally without judging them).

What the Science says about the Effectiveness of Meditation?

Many studies have investigated meditation for different conditions, and there's evidence that it may reduce blood pressure as well as symptoms of irritable bowel syndrome and flare-ups in people who have had ulcerative colitis. It may ease symptoms of anxiety and depression, and may help people with insomnia.

Meditation helps with these conditions:

- Pain,
- For High Blood Pressure,
- For Irritable Bowel Syndrome,
- For Ulcerative Colitis,
- For Anxiety, Depression, and Insomnia,
- For Smoking Cessation,
- Other Conditions.

Meditation and the Brain

Some research suggests that meditation may physically change the brain and body and could potentially help to improve many health problems and promote healthy behaviors.

Safety and Side Effects

- Meditation is generally considered to be safe for healthy people.
- People with physical limitations may not be able to participate in certain meditative practices involving movement. People with physical health conditions should speak with their health care providers before starting a meditative practice, and make their meditation instructor aware of their condition.
- There have been rare reports that meditation could cause or worsen symptoms in people with certain psychiatric problems like anxiety and depression. People with existing mental health conditions should speak with their health care providers before starting a meditative practice, and make their meditation instructor aware of their condition.

References

- Brief presurgery hypnosis reduces distress and pain in excisional breast biopsy patients. Int J Clin Exp Hypn. 2002;50:17-32
- Sadock BJ, Sadock VA, eds. Kaplan & Sadock's Comprehensive Textbook of Psychiatry. Vol 2. 7th ed. Philadelphia, Pa: Lippincott Williams & Wilkins; 2000:2138- 2146

- Mindbody-medicine, encyclopedias-almanacs-transcripts-and-maps: encyclopedia.com, Retrieved 10 March, 2019
- Where the imaginal appears real: a positron emission tomography study of auditory hallucinations. Proc Natl Acad Sci U S A. 1998;95:1956-1960
- Suggestion, relaxation, and hypnosis as adjuncts in the care of surgery patients: a review of the literature. Am J Clin Hypn. 1991; 33:172-186

4

Common Alternative Therapies

Alternative therapies are gaining popularity across the globe. Some of the common alternative therapies such as aromatherapy, reflexology, chiropractic, reiki, shiatsu, etc. have been carefully analyzed in this chapter.

Aromatherapy

Aromatherapy is the practice of using volatile plant oils, including essential oils, for psychological and physical well-being. Essential oils, the pure essence of a plant, have been found to provide both psychological and physical benefits when used correctly and safely.

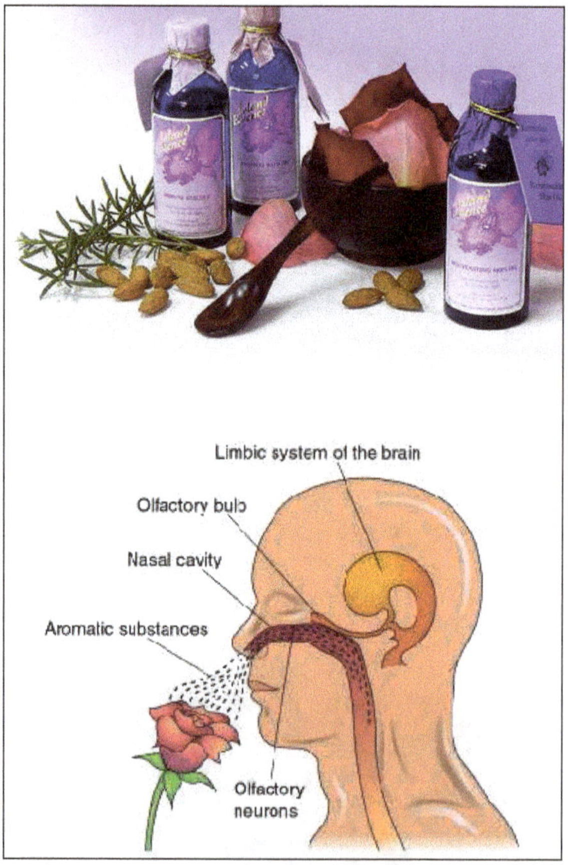

Aromatherapy.

The Essential Oil Profiles area details over 90 essential oils. Absolutes, CO_2 and Hydrosols are also commonly utilized in aromatherapy. Although essential oils, CO_2 extracts and absolutes are distilled by different methods, the term essential oil is sometimes used as a blanket term to include all natural, aromatic, volatile, plant oils including CO_2 and absolutes. In addition to essential oils, aromatherapy encourages the use of other complementary natural ingredients including cold pressed vegetable oils, jojoba (a liquid wax), hydrosols, herbs, milk powders, sea salts, sugars (an exfoliant), clays and muds. Products that include synthetic ingredients are frowned upon in holistic aromatherapy. It is important to note that perfume oils also known as fragrance oils (and usually listed as "fragrance" on an ingredient label) are not the same as essential oils. Fragrance oils and perfume oils contain synthetic chemicals and do not provide the therapeutic benefits of essential oils.

The Benefit of an Aroma – Inhaling Essential

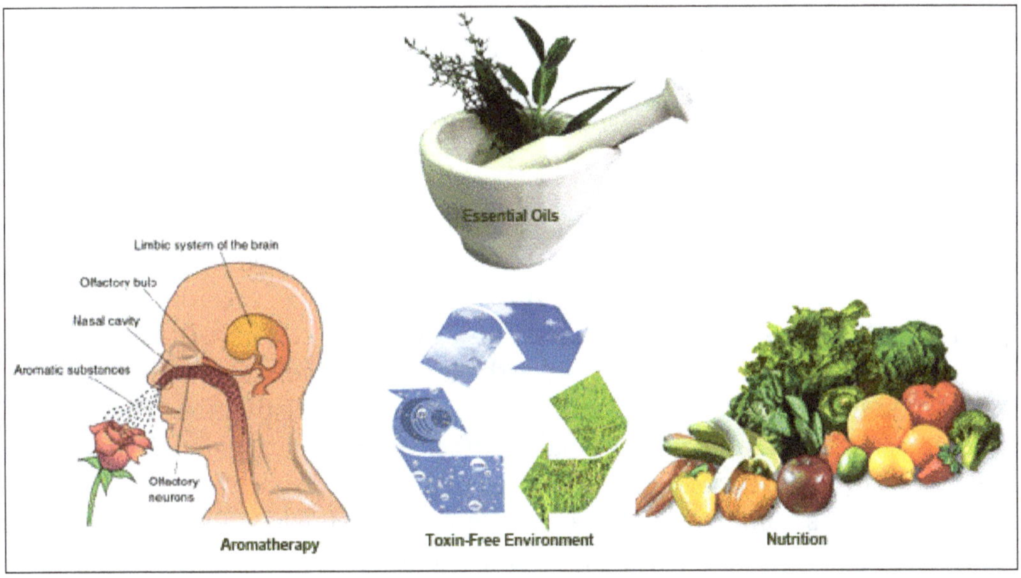

Aroma from essential oils.

- Oils: Essential oils that are inhaled into the lungs offer both psychological and physical benefits. Not only does the aroma of the natural essential oil stimulate the brain to trigger a reaction, but when inhaled into the lungs, the natural constituents (naturally occurring chemicals) can supply therapeutic benefit. Diffusing eucalyptus essential oil to help ease congestion is a prominent example. If not done correctly and safely, however, the use of essential oils can have severe consequences.
- The Benefit of Physical Application: Essential oils that are applied to the skin can be absorbed into the bloodstream. The constituents of essential oils can aid in health, beauty and hygiene conditions. Since essential oils are so powerful and concentrated, they should never be applied to the skin in their undiluted

form. To apply essential oils to the skin, essential oils are typically diluted into a carrier such as a cold pressed vegetable oil, also known as a carrier oil. Common carrier oils include sweet almond oil, apricot kernel oil and grapeseed oil. A more detailed definition of Carrier Oils is found on the what are Carrier Oils page. A detailed list of carrier oils and their properties can be found on the Carrier Oils Used in Aromatherapy properties page.

- Other Benefits: In addition to therapeutic benefit at the emotional and physical level, essential oils are helpful in other applications. Essential oils can be used in household and laundry cleaners. Some oils act as a natural insect repellent and pesticide. You may recall using citronella candles during the summer to keep mosquitoes away. Citronella essential oil is the ingredient in the candles that is responsible for repelling the mosquitos.

- Essential Oil Blends: Essential oils can be blended together to create appealing and complex aromas. Essential oils can also be blended for a specific therapeutic application. Essential oils that are carefully blended with a specific therapeutic purpose in mind may be referred to as an essential oil syngery. A synergistic essential oil blend is considered to be greater in total action than each oil working independently.

Aromatherapy may have origins in antiquity with the use of infused aromatic oils, made by macerating dried plant material in fatty oil, heating and then filtering. Many such oils are described by Dioscorides, along with beliefs of the time regarding their healing properties, in his De Materia Medica, written in the first century. Distilled essential oils have been employed as medicines since the invention of distillation in the eleventh century, when Avicenna isolated essential oils using steam distillation. The concept of aromatherapy was first mooted by a small number of European scientists and doctors, in about 1907. In 1937, the word first appeared in print in a French book on the subject: Aromathérapie: Les Huiles Essentielles, Hormones Végétales by RenéMaurice Gattefossé, a chemist. An English version was published in 1993. In 1910, Gattefossé burned a hand very badly in a laboratory explosion. The hand developed gas gangrene, which he successfully, and intentionally, treated with lavender oil.

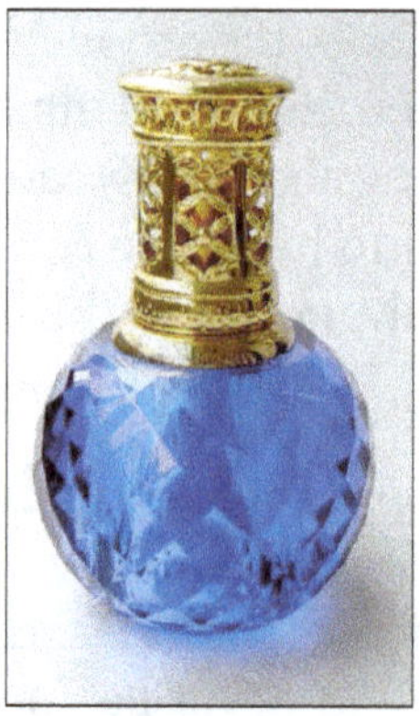

A French surgeon, Jean Valnet, pioneered the medicinal uses of essential oils, which he used as antiseptics in the treatment of wounded soldiers during World War II.

Modes of Application

The modes of application of aromatherapy include:

- Aerial diffusion: For environmental fragrancing or aerial disinfection.
- Direct inhalation: For respiratory disinfection, decongestion, expectoration as well as psychological effects.
- Topical applications: For general massage, baths, compresses, therapeutic skin care.
- Materials.

Some of the materials employed include:

- Absolutes: Fragrant oils extracted primarily from flowers or delicate plant tissues through solvent or supercritical fluid extraction (e.g., rose absolute). The term is also used to describe oils extracted from fragrant butters, concretes, and enfleurage pommades using ethanol.
- Carrier oils: Typically oily plant base triacylglycerides that dilute essential oils for use on the skin (e.g., sweet almond oil).
- Essential oils: Fragrant oils extracted from plants chiefly through steam distillation (e.g., eucalyptus oil) or expression (grapefruit oil). However, the term is also occasionally used to describe fragrant oils extracted from plant material by any solvent extraction.
- Herbal distillates or hydrosols: The aqueous byproducts of the distillation process (e.g., rosewater). There are many herbs that make herbal distillates and they have culinary uses, medicinal uses and skin care uses. Common herbal distillates are chamomile, rose, and lemon balm.
- Infusions: Aqueous extracts of various plant materials (e.g., infusion of chamomile).
- Phytoncides: Various volatile organic compounds from plants that kill microbes. Many terpenebased fragrant oils and sulfuric compounds from plants in the genus "Allium" are phytoncides, though the latter are likely less commonly used in aromatherapy due to their disagreeable odors.
- Vaporizer (volatized) raw herbs: Typically higher oil content plant based materials dried, crushed, and heated to extract and inhale the aromatic oil vapors in a direct inhalation modality.

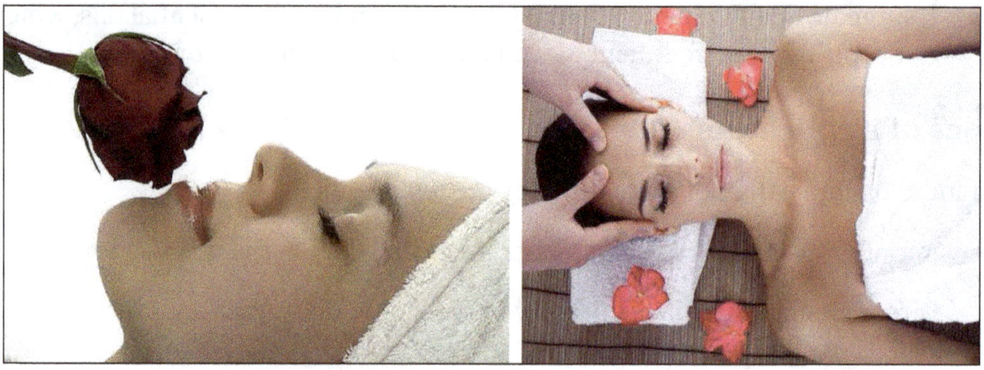

Aromatherapy for altering a person's mind, mood, cognitive function or health.

Theory

Aromatherapy is the treatment or prevention of disease by use of essential oils. Other stated uses include pain and anxiety reduction, enhancement of energy and short-term memory, relaxation, hair loss prevention, and reduction of eczema-induced itching. Two basic mechanisms are offered to explain the purported effects. One is the influence of aroma on the brain, especially the limbic system through the olfactory system. The other is the direct pharmacological effects of the essential oils.3 While precise knowledge of the synergy between the body and aromatic oils is often claimed by aromatherapists, the efficacy of aromatherapy remains unproven. However, some preliminary clinical studies of aromatherapy in combination with other techniques show positive effects. Aromatherapy does not cure conditions, but helps the body to find a natural way to cure itself and improve immune response.

Applied Kinesiology

Applied kinesiology (AK) is the study of muscles and the relationship of muscle strength to health. It incorporates a system of manual muscle testing and therapy. AK is based on the theory that an organ dysfunction is accompanied by a specific muscle weakness. Diseases are diagnosed through muscle-testing procedures and then treated. AK is not the same as kinesiology, or biomechanics, which is the scientific study of movement.

Origins

AK is based on principles of functional neurology, anatomy, physiology, biomechanics, and biochemistry as well as principles from Chinese medicine, acupuncture, and massage. It was developed from traditional kinesiology in 1964 by George G. Goodheart, a chiropractor from Detroit, Michigan. He observed that each large muscle relates to a body organ. A weakness in a muscle may mean that there is a problem in the associated organ. Goodheart found that by treating the muscle and making it strong again, he was able to improve the function of the organ as well. For example, if a particular nutritional supplement was given to a patient, and the muscle tested strong, it was the correct supplement for the patient. If the muscle remained weak, it was not. Other methods of treatment can be evaluated in a similar manner. Goodheart also found that painful nodules (small bumps) may be associated with a weak muscle. By deeply massaging the muscle, he was able to improve its strength. Goodheart's findings in 1964 led to the origin and insertion treatment, the first method developed in AK. Other diagnostic and therapeutic procedures were developed for various reflexes described by other chiropractors and doctors. Goodheart incorporated acupuncture meridian therapy into AK after reading the writings of Felix Mann, M.D.

Goodheart considered AK to be a therapeutic tool that incorporates feedback from the body. He said that "applied kinesiology is based on the fact that the body language never lies." He felt that the body's muscles were indicators of disharmony. Once muscle weakness has been ascertained, the problem may be solved in a variety of ways. If a practitioner approaches the problem correctly, he believed, making the proper and adequate diagnosis and treatment, the outcome is satisfactory both to the doctor and to the patient.

Benefits

AK is not designed for crisis medicine. For example, an AK practitioner cannot cure cancer, arthritis, diabetes, heart disease, or infections . This therapy is designed to be a part of a holistic approach to preventive medicine. The goals of AK are to (1) restore normal nerve function, (2) achieve normal endocrine, immune, digestive, and other internal organ functions, (3) intervene early in degenerative processes to prevent or delay pathological conditions, and to (4) restore postural balance, correct gait (walking) impairment, and improve range of motion.

According to AK, each muscle in the body relates to a specific meridian or energy pathway (acupuncture lines) in the body. These meridians also relate to organs or glands, allowing the muscles to provide information about organ or gland function and energy. The five areas of diagnosis and therapy for the applied kinesiologist are (1) the nervous system, (2) the lymphatic system, (3) the vascular (blood vessel) system, (4) the cerebrospinal system, and (5) the meridian system.

The first part of AK is muscle testing, which is used to help diagnose what part of the body is functioning abnormally. Muscle testing involves putting the body into a position that requires a certain muscle to remain contracted, and then applying pressure against the muscle. The testing does not measure strength but is meant to reveal stresses and imbalances in the body through the tension in the muscle. The test evaluates the ability of a controlling system to adapt the muscle to meet the changing pressure of the examiner's test. AK practitioners also examine structural factors such as posture, gait, and range of motion. Some chiropractors use AK to help them evaluate the success of spinal adjustment. A leg muscle is tested for strength or weakness to determine whether the adjustments made are appropriate.

According to AK, common internal causes of muscle weakness include:

- Dysfunction of nerve supply (nerve interference between spine and muscles).
- Impairment of lymphatic drainage.
- Reduction of blood supply.
- Abnormal pressure in cerebral fluid affecting nerve-to-muscle relationships.
- Blockage of an acupuncture meridian.
- Imbalance of chemicals.
- Dysfunction of organs or glands.
- Excesses or deficiencies in nutrition.

Physiological reactions to chemicals, including those associated with nutrition and allergies , may also be evaluated using AK. The AK protocol for testing chemical compounds is to place the substance on the patient's tongue so that he tastes the material, and the normal chemical reactions of ingestion begin. In some cases, the substances are inhaled through the nose. The AK practitioner then tests the associated muscle-organ pattern to determine where or if there is a strength or weakness. The patient does not need to swallow the substance for a change in strength or weakness to be identified. David S. Walther, a diplomate of the International College of Applied Kinesiology, has indicated that "it is possible that the central nervous system, recognizing the compound being ingested, relays information to the organs and glands preparing for use of the compound. If the compound is recognized as beneficial, the energy pattern is immediately enhanced, influencing not only the organ or gland, but also the associated muscle."

AK has been used as a diagnostic health tool for a variety of conditions.

Bone health:

- Neck/low back pain and sciatica,
- Whiplash,
- Frozen shoulder.

Joint health:

- Carpal tunnel syndrome,

- Arthritis (including rheumatoid arthritis),
- Sports injuries.

Chelation Therapy

Chelation therapy, a program of repeated intravenous administration of ethylene diamine tetraacetic acid (EDTA), often given in combination with vitamins and minerals, has been touted as a safe alternative treatment for atherosclerotic vascular disease. As this is a non-conventional therapy, there is no universally recognized standard protocol. Most protocols, however, share a degree of similarity. A typical protocol might consist of 30intravenously administered solutions of 3 grams of disodium EDTA with concomitant administration of varying levels of ascorbic acid, B-vitamins, heparin, and the minerals magnesium, copper, zinc, selenium and manganese delivered over 1.5 to 3 hours in 500 ml to 1000 ml of normal saline. Therapy is often delivered on a weekly or biweekly basis and may be followed up with a less frequent maintenance schedule.

There is a very strong market for this therapy with out-of-pocket costs for the use of EDTA to treat cardiovascular disease estimated to range from $400 million to $3 billion annually in the United States. The use of chelation therapy for cardiovascular disease appears to contradict conventional medical thought, however, as three systematic reviews of clinical trials have concluded that chelation therapy is not supported by the evidence. In contrast, one early meta-analysis of uncontrolled trials and unpublished data claimed that EDTA chelation therapy effectively improved the symptoms of cardiovascular disease in over 80% of cases.

There is continued controversy as to the use of this therapy and a substantial amount of press given to it in popular non-peer reviewed literature and on the Internet.

Chiropractic

Chiropractic is an important component of the US health care system and the largest alternative medical profession. In this overview of chiropractic, we examine its history, theory, and development; its scientific evidence; and its approach to the art of medicine. Chiropractic's position in society is contradictory, and we reveal a complex dynamic of conflict and diversity. Internally, chiropractic has a dramatic legacy of strife and factionalism. Externally, it has defended itself from vigorous opposition by conventional medicine. Despite such tensions, chiropractors have maintained a unified profession with an uninterrupted commitment to clinical care. While the core chiropractic belief that the correction of spinal abnormality is a critical health care intervention is open to debate, chiropractic's most important contribution may have to do with the patient-physician relationship.

Chiropractic, the medical profession that specializes in manual therapy and especially spinal manipulation, is the most important example of alternative medicine in the United States and alternative medicine's greatest anomaly.

Even to call chiropractic "alternative" is problematic; in many ways, it is distinctly mainstream. Facts such as the following attest to its status and success: Chiropractic is licensed in all 50 states. An estimated 1 of 3 persons with lower back pain is treated by chiropractors. In 1988 (the latest year with reliable statistics), between $2.4 and $4 billion was spent on chiropractic care, and in 1990, 160 million office visits were made to chiropractors. Since 1972, Medicare has reimbursed patients for chiropractic treatments, and these treatments are covered as well by most major insurance companies. In 1994, the Agency for Health Care Policy and Research removed much of the onus of marginality from chiropractic by declaring that spinal manipulation can alleviate low back pain. In addition, the profession is growing: the number of chiropractors in the United States—now at 50,000—is expected to double by 2010 (whereas the number of physicians is expected to increase by only 16%).

Despite such impressive credentials, academic medicine regards chiropractic theory as speculative at best and its claims of clinical success, at least outside of low back pain, as unsubstantiated. Only a few small hospitals permit chiropractors to treat inpatients, and to our knowledge, university-affiliated teaching centers have not yet granted chiropractors privileges to perform manipulation on patients. Although the American Medical Association (AMA) no longer prohibits its members from consulting with chiropractors, especially since it was found guilty of conspiracy in this regard, chiropractic's size and power have not translated into complete acceptance.

Contradictions and tensions exist not only between chiropractic and mainstream medicine but within chiropractic itself. Since its inception, chiropractors have disagreed about the definition of the therapy and its scope of practice. Various theories vie for dominance within the profession. A multiplicity of competing adjustment techniques also vie with each other under the rubric of chiropractic. The mode of chiropractic intervention—by means of the hands—and its unique therapeutic niche, primarily pain disorders, seem too narrow a foundation for its claim to encompass a distinct health system with autonomous licensing, credentialing, and educational institutions.

Yet, despite external conflicts and perhaps partly because of them, and despite the intraprofessional disagreements and uncertainty about its scope of practice, chiropractic has found an internal coherence that has allowed it to become an enduring presence in the United States. This integrity has to do with the profession's belief in the importance of biomechanics; the centrality of manual therapy, especially for the spine; and a clinical dynamic that provides patients with explanations, meaning, and concrete experiences that promote a strong patient-physician bond, a sense of caring, and a restored sense of well-being.

Chiropractic's Origin

Most sources date the birth of chiropractic as September 18, 1895, when Daniel David (usually called "D.D.") Palmer shoved a single cervical vertebra of a deaf janitor of the Putnam Building in downtown Davenport, Iowa. A mythic aura clings to the event, partly because of its importance and because there is little agreement among witnesses about when it happened, who was there, or what actually occurred. (The mythic aspect of the story may have been intentionally enhanced by selecting the date of Rosh Hashanah, the Jewish New Year, which was an occasion for revelation in 19th-century American millennialism. Whether fact, folklore, or both, the founding blow of chiropractic was more than a chance event or momentary inspiration. In fact, it creatively synthesized 4 previously distinct health care traditions: bonesetting, magnetic healing, orthodox science, and popular health reform.

Bonesetters

Bonesetters were a common fixture in 19th-century health care. As with the other healing crafts—midwifery, tooth-pulling, and barber-surgery—bonesetting was often part-time work and served clients who had problems that were regarded by academically trained physicians as inconsequential or beneath their dignity. Bonesetters did much more than help mend bones. They often treated painful conditions caused by "subluxations," which meant a "joint 'put out'; and the one method of cure is the wrench aid, the rough movement by which it is said that the joint is 'put in' again."

Palmer frequently mentioned the bonesetter's tradition, identified with it, and probably had some training in it. Palmer's innovation professionalized the craft, guaranteeing its continuation into the modern era. The upgrade extended to nomenclature; with help from a minister conversant with Greek, "bonesetting" became "chiropractic," a phrase that means "hand work."

Magnetic Healing

Although the bonesetting tradition gave chiropractic its method, "magnetic healing" provided the theory. Palmer acknowledged a special debt to magnetic healing when he wrote, "chiropractic was not evolved from medicine or any other method, except that of magnetic."(p111) Derived from Anton Mesmer's (1734-1815) investigations into the supposed curative effects of animal magnetism, practitioners of magnetic healing identified the unimpeded flow of energy with health and defined illness as obstruction. For 9 years before his discovery of chiropractic, Palmer was one of a small army of healers who routinely "magnetized" their patients. Palmer's major revision of traditional magnetism was to call it "innate intelligence" and to claim that its pathway was the human nervous system, especially the spinal cord. Misaligned spinal vertebrae (the redefined bonesetters' "subluxation") impinge on this beneficent flow and cause illness. By marrying magnetism to bonesetting, Palmer created a new and independent medical movement, one more capable of competing for legitimacy than either of its predecessors had been.

Neither bonesetting nor magnetic healing could be persuasively described as science. The former was clearly a folk tradition, and the latter could not shed its occult status. Chiropractic, however, could and did describe itself as science, and in the 19th century, such a label was indispensable if a medical movement hoped to emerge from a host of contending traditions. Although self-taught, Palmer saw himself as a scientist and wasted no time in adopting prevailing scientific notions of the spinal cord to chiropractic theory. An early 19th-century fascination with the spinal cord led to mainstream speculation, and by 1828, orthodox physicians began to warn about the threat posed to the organs of the body by "spinal irritation." Spinal irritation in the 19th century became a catchall for a host of complaints. The theory was so well accepted that Oliver Wendell Holmes (1809-1894) could comfortably tell the 1871 graduating class of Bellevue Hospital College that he kept the phrase "spinal irritation" "on hand for patients that sic will insist on knowing the pathology of their complaints." Gradually discarded by mainstream medicine and replaced by the term "neurasthenia" (and later, "depression"), spinal irritation entered into chiropractic through the subluxation terminology of bonesetters. Palmer extended the scope of spinal irritation and subluxation beyond the class of ailments that otherwise defied analysis; it was, for him, the key to understanding sickness as a whole. At the same time, the adoption of the widely accepted concept of spinal irritation lent credibility to chiropractic.

Popular Health Reform

Palmer cured the Davenport janitor of his deafness. This restoration of hearing might have been regarded as a freak occurrence were it not for a medical environment in which news of such occurrences was eagerly awaited. A well-publicized tug-of-war between "regulars" (physicians) and "irregulars" (alternative medicine practitioners) already had been sweeping the country. The introduction of homeopathy, herbal medicine, "Mind Cure," Christian Science, health food, and hydropathy had prepared Americans to look for cases that, on the one hand, pointed to the limitations of mainstream medicine and, on the other, made the miraculous seem obtainable. The way to perfect health was on the horizon, waiting to be grasped, described, and disseminated.

The unique union of bonesetting, magnetism, and orthodoxy was warmly received. The conflict for medical hegemony both helped and was helped by chiropractic. Palmer's invectives against the establishment of "germo-anti-toxis-vaxi-radi-electro-microbio-slush death producers" resonated with the movement, as did his grandiose promises of a medicine "destined to be the grandest and greatest of this or any age" because it was successful in all forms of disease. Chiropractic was the glamorous new recruit in the old war with mainstream medicine.

Spinal Manipulation: The Core Chiropractic Act

Adjusting with the hands—the signature chiropractic gesture—is the unifying activity that allows chiropractic to transcend its internal discord and create a coherent profession. Overriding disputes within the profession, the core question for all chiropractors remains unchanged and agreed on: how should the hands move the vertebrae? Beneath doctrinal disparity and clinical diversity, chiropractic has an internal cohesion that is more than a defensive reaction to a critical world. Chiropractors believe that the correction of spinal abnormality—the adjustment of vertebrae—is a critical healing act.

Obviously, vertebrae move all the time. The physical activities of daily life—exercise, turning, twisting, bending—require a normal range of motion. Greater mobility, or "mobilization," can be coaxed from the joints with the assistance of a physical therapist, for example, who can stretch the lower spine by gently moving the thigh of a person lying on his or her side. Eventually, mobilization reaches an elastic barrier of resistance, known to chiropractors as "end feel."

Chiropractic manipulation is a method of moving vertebrae beyond end feel, but not so far as to destroy the integrity of joint structure. The adjustment temporarily creates an increased range of motion. The patient feels the change and often hears a popping or cracking noise, which some attribute to a sudden liberation of synovial gases.

The vertebrae can be moved by direct contact—the "short-lever" technique—or through a distant linkage, or the "long-lever" method. The latter method is used, for example, when a dynamic thrust of the thigh moves a vertebra in the lower spine. "Amplitude" refers to the depth or distance traveled by a practitioner's thrust. When joints are less accessible or when a long lever is involved, the amplitude increases. The degree of force applied is yet another variable.

Emblematic Chiropractic Adjustment

Palmer claimed to have discovered the use of spinous and transverse processes of the spine as levers and to be the first to use direct contact with a vertebra that was "out." B. J. Palmer developed the "recoil adjustment," in which a practitioner quickly pushes the vertebra into motion and then, instead of maintaining pressure, relies on a fast release to generate a type of rebound. B. J. Palmer thought this maneuver allowed the body's innate intelligence to set a vertebra in its exact place. With or without recoil adjustment, the short-lever technique—touching the vertebra directly at high velocity and low amplitude, that is, by moving a small distance—with the spinal or transverse process as a fulcrum is considered the typical chiropractic maneuver.

Diversity in Manipulation

Chiropractors besides the Palmers were quick to make their own contributions, and the profession soon encompassed diverse styles, which often occasioned fresh disputes. Whereas the Palmers emphasized one vertebra at a time, Carver developed methods to adjust the lumbar spine as a unit. Practitioners such as Oakley Smith and Solon Langworthy borrowed long-lever osteopathic techniques and folk methods such as Bohemian (Czech) manipulation. "Diversified technique" is the label for the largest and most eclectic collection of different methods many chiropractors use.

Besides the forceful techniques, gentler methods of manipulation are common in chiropractic. The sacro-occipital technique, developed by DeJarnette in the 1930s, relies on the passive weight of a patient pressing down on strategically placed padded wedges to reposition the pelvis and spine. The Logan basic technique applies light thumb pressure close to the sacrotuberous ligament to move the sacrum. The activator technique makes use of a small spring-loaded instrument that looks like a small plunger with a hard sponge on the tip to deliver pressure to the vertebrae. Some practitioners use tables with segmental drop pieces to allow low-force, high-velocity adjustment. In total, observers of the profession have counted between 96 and more than 200 specifically chiropractic-type maneuvers. Most chiropractors draw on a variety of maneuvers on the basis of education and personal affinity, and most develop their own distinctive style.

Chiropractic Health Care

Chiropractic health care is based on the endemic presence of pain, especially low back pain, in the United States. Between 70% and 80% of all adults experience low back pain at some time in their lives, and in any one year, more than 50% of Americans suffer from the telltale nagging-tugging sensation. So pervasive is back pain in this society that, as one authority has mused, it might be abnormal not to suffer from it. Chronic pain is no less a problem, and data suggest that nearly a third of the American population suffers from some sort of chronic pain.

It is no secret that low back pain and chronic pain are the Achilles' heel of biomedicine and present a need and opportunity for alternative responses. By far the largest percentage of patients—at least 80%—go to chiropractors for neuroskeletal and musculoskeletal problems. Of these patients, at least 65% have back pain; most other symptoms involve the neck, extremities, and head.

Patient Perceptions

Many large and methodologically sound surveys from diverse sampling populations leave little doubt that patients believe chiropractic works for them. The results show that most chiropractic patients and former patients are likely to be satisfied with the treatment they received. Studies that compare patients' satisfaction with chiropractic with that of conventional medicine in treating low back pain demonstrate marked preference for chiropractic. A 1986 survey of members of a Washington State health maintenance organization that offers both conventional and chiropractic care compared the responses of 359 patients treated by conventional physicians with those of 348 patients treated by chiropractors. Patients treated by chiropractors for low back pain were 3 times as likely—66% to 22%—to report that they were "very satisfied" with the care they had received. A Utah study (1973) reported comparable results. Patients perceive chiropractic as a valuable component of their health care.

Diet Therapy

Diet therapy, an alternative therapy uses specialized dietary regimens (such as the macrobiotic, Paleo, Mediterranean, and low carbohydrate diets) to:

- Treat or prevent a specific disease (such as cancer or cardiovascular disorders).
- Generally promote wellness.
- Detoxify the body (by neutralizing or eliminating toxins from the body).

Some diets (such as the Mediterranean diet) are widely accepted and encouraged in traditional.

Western Medicine

When beginning a therapeutic diet that involves a dramatically different way of eating, people should ask an expert to advise them so that they can avoid nutritional deficiencies. Dietary science and understanding is constantly evolving and should be revisited frequently with a healthcare or nutrition professional.

Macrobiotic Diet

The macrobiotic diet consists of largely vegetables, whole grains, fruits, and cereals. Some people following a macrobiotic diet have reported improvements in cancer and its symptoms, but well-designed studies have not shown this.

Risks of a macrobiotic diet include unintended weight loss and sometimes inadequate intake of certain nutrients.

Paleo Diet

The Paleo diet consists of types of food allegedly consumed in the distant past during the Paleolithic (Stone Age) era, when food was hunted or gathered. That is, it consists of foods made from animals and wild plants. Thus, the diet results in the following:

- Eating more protein.
- Eating fewer carbohydrates and, when eating them, eating mainly nonstarchy fresh fruits and vegetables.
- Consuming more fiber.
- Often eating more fat, mainly monounsaturated and polyunsaturated fats.

Foods thought not to be available during the Paleolithic era (such as dairy products, grains, legumes, processed oils, refined sugar, salt, and coffee) are avoided. Proponents claim that people cannot process (metabolize) many of these foods. However, knowledge of what was eaten in the Paleolithic era is limited, and some evidence suggests that in the Paleolithic era, the diet was not as limited as the modern Paleo diet.

Proponents of the Paleo diet claim that it reduces the risk of coronary artery disease, type 2 diabetes, and many chronic conditions. They also claim it promotes weight loss, improves athletic performance, enhances sleep, and improves mental function. However, evidence that this diet has any of these effects remains inconsistent.

Risks of the Paleo diet include inadequate intake of certain nutrients (due to decreased consumption of whole grains and dairy products) and possibly an increased risk of coronary artery disease (due to increased consumption of fat and protein).

Energy Therapy

Energy therapies are alternative therapies that aim to create a state of balance, health and peace in a person. An underlying theory to energy therapies involves energy blockages or imbalances that lead to illness and disease. The most popular forms of energy therapy are music therapy, Therapeutic Touch and Reiki.

All energy therapies are considered complements — not replacements — to traditional cancer treatment. Energy therapies cannot cure or directly treat cancer. These therapies can help people relax and may improve quality of life among people with mesothelioma and other cancers.

When people talk about energy in energy medicine, they are usually referring to an energy field or form of energy that hasn't been proven to exist. The National Center for

Complementary and Alternative Medicine (NCCAM) distinguishes proven energy from the unproven. NCCAM uses two classifications:

- Verifiable energy is measurable and scientifically proven.
- Unverifiable energy is not measurable with current technology and may not exist.

Examples of verifiable energy include sound energy (vibration), electromagnetic energy (such as light), magnetism and monochromatic radiation (lasers).

Doctors regularly use verifiable energy to diagnose and treat cancer. Examples include magnetic resonance imaging (MRI), lasers used during surgery, radiation therapy and photodynamic therapy. Less-researched therapies in this category include magnetic therapy and sound energy therapy.

Traditional doctors do not use unverifiable energy in medical practice. Energy therapies are primarily available through alternative medicine practitioners.

How Does it Work?

Therapies based on unverifiable energy, such as Reiki and Therapeutic Touch, reflect the belief that people possess a subtle form of life-force energy that isn't measurable by modern science. This subtle, unproven energy is often called qi in traditional Chinese medicine, prana in ayurvedic medicine and spirit in Judeo-Christian traditions. Some people refer to it as vital life-force energy or the bioenergetic field (which often gets confused with bioenergetic exchanges, the transfer of verifiable energy among organisms and their environment).

Balancing this proposed life-force energy is the goal of energy therapies. The same goal is shared by more popular mind-body therapies (yoga, qigong and tai chi) and certain healing systems, such as Ayurveda and traditional Chinese medicine. Acupuncture is also based on the belief of life-force energy. However, current research is finding plausible biological explanations for the health effects of acupuncture.

Some scientists propose that verifiable energy may be the only energy at play when therapeutic benefit is experienced through energy therapy.

Whether a subtle, separate energy exists does not change the fact that many people feel therapeutic benefits from energy therapies. The placebo effect may be at play. Since a placebo has a measurable effect in many scientific studies, many people believe that energy therapies can help people with cancer regardless of lacking evidence for life-force energy.

Various physiological actions might underlie the benefits of energy therapies. For example, acupuncture and acupressure points are often located at sites with a high density of nerve and blood vessels, commonly between or at the edges of muscle groups. Stimulation of these areas has physiological effects on the nervous system, musculoskeletal system and endocrine system. The effects of touch, which stimulate the release of feel-good chemicals, such as oxytocin in the brain, might also play a role.

Sound Therapies

Music therapy and sound energy therapy are two types of sound therapy that may benefit people with cancer.

Music Therapy

Music therapy is the use of music by trained professionals to encourage relaxation and enhance quality of life in people receiving health care. The hope is to relieve stress and promote well-being. Some people experience reduction of symptoms and improved healing.

Trained music therapists tailor sessions to individuals and groups based on their needs and musical preferences. A session may involve listening to music, making music, writing songs and discussing lyrics. Music therapy is given in various settings like hospitals, treatment centers, at home or outdoors. Patients do not need any musical ability to experience or benefit from music therapy.

Music therapy can ease nausea and vomiting following high-dose chemotherapy when combined with anti-nausea drugs. In people with cancer, music therapy can:

- Provide comfort and relaxation.
- Reduce short-term pain.
- Decrease intensity of pain when combined with pain-reducing drugs.
- Minimize the need for pain medication in some patients.
- Improve quality of life.

Other studies on music therapy show that it may reduce breathing rate, heart rate, blood pressure, insomnia, depression and anxiety. Music therapy can also affect stress hormones and brain waves (which can induce relaxation). A handful of studies on neurologic music therapy report that it eases depression, improves stuttering, enhances brain plasticity, and improves function and emotional adjustment in people with traumatic brain injury.

This therapy is not based on unverifiable energy. The benefits of music therapy come from the psychological effects of listening to music you like and connecting with other people in a therapeutic setting.

Sound Energy Therapy

Sound energy therapy uses instruments or pre-recorded tones to produce sounds that soothe listeners into a state of relaxation. Instruments commonly used during sound energy therapy sessions include Tibetan singing bowls, crystal bowls and tuning forks.

Pre-recorded sounds are often designed to deliver two tones at a different frequency into each ear. This causes the listener to perceive a single tone that varies in amplitude at a frequency equal to the difference between the two tones. The single tone perceived by the brain is known as a binaural auditory beat.

These types of sound therapy haven't been as thoroughly researched as music therapy. Though few clinical studies have scientifically investigated sound energy therapy, people say it promotes deep relaxation, enhances learning, improves sleep and reduces perception of stress. Studies on binaural auditory beat suggest it may improve sleep, memory task performance, attention, relaxation and mood.

Touch Therapies

In some energy therapies, practitioners use gentle touch or hover their hands over the patient with the intention of sending energy into the body or balancing energy within the body. Proponents say the benefits of these therapies are a result of enhancing or balancing life-force energy. Others suggest the benefits are a result of factors surrounding the experience, such as the biological effects of touch and the psychological effects of the health care experience.

Reiki

Reiki is a therapeutic practice based on the idea that a person's life-force energy can be cleansed, rejuvenated and balanced by transferring energy through the hands of a trained practitioner. A Reiki practitioner places their hands in more than a dozen positions on or over a patient's body to transfer energy. Proponents say the energy can be sent from a distance as well.

The exact history of Reiki is unclear. It likely originated in Japan, possibly with a man named Dr. Mikao Usui around the early 1900s. Hawayo Takata, a female student of Usui's style of Reiki, brought the teachings to the United States in the late 1930s. Today, roughly one million Americans receive Reiki every year.

Limited clinical research has been conducted on Reiki. Most of the research is anecdotal or qualitative rather than quantitative, meaning the studies are usually based upon participants' reports and rarely on randomized, controlled scientific studies. Anecdotal reports show that people who receive Reiki often feel more relaxed, with reduced stress and increased well-being. One small, controlled pilot study found Reiki helped to reduce cancer patients' self-reports of pain, but did not reduce their need for pain-reducing medication.

Even though clinical studies cannot find strong evidence to support Reiki, many people who receive Reiki tout the relaxing and healing effects of the therapy.

Therapeutic Touch

Therapeutic Touch (TT) is similar to Reiki in that a trained practitioner uses his or her hands to send healing energy to a person. This therapy was developed in the early 1970s by Delores Krieger, Ph.D., R.N., a professor of nursing at New York University, and Dora Kunz, a natural healer. Proponents of TT claim the therapy can reduce anxiety, improve healing and treat numerous ailments, from headaches to nausea to cancer.

Thousands of nurses throughout the United States and Canada are trained in Therapeutic Touch. During a TT session, a practitioner senses blockages in a patient's life-force energy field and sends healing energy through his or her hands to clear blockages or harmful energy.

A scientific review of 83 studies on TT found only one study that may have independently confirmed a positive effect.

The review also included a study to determine whether trained TT practitioners could identify which of their hands was closest to an investigator's hand under blinded conditions to prove they could sense another person's energy. Out of 21 practitioners with experience ranging from one to 27 years, none could correctly and repeatedly identify the location of an investigator's hand. Overall, the practitioners identified the correct hand in 123 of 280 trials. The investigators state this 44 percent success rate is consistent with random chance.

The investigators concluded that the experienced TT practitioners could not detect an investigator's energy field. They stated that the "failure to substantiate TT's most fundamental claim is unrefuted evidence that the claims of TT are groundless."

Regardless of the lack of scientific evidence for Therapeutic Touch, many nurses use the therapy, and patients continue to report benefits from TT sessions.

Spiritual Healing

Spiritual healing is similar to touch therapies in that spiritual healers believe they can channel energy into a client's body to promote healing. However, spiritual healing doesn't necessarily involve touch and practitioners say it can be performed from a great distance. Spiritual healing is also called intercessory prayer or faith, psychic or distant healing.

Reviews of more than 20 randomized clinical trials of spiritual healing have found no evidence that it helps people recover from cancer or any other ailment.

Electromagnetic Field Therapy

Electromagnetic field therapy uses electromagnetic energy generated by an electric current to treat pain or illness. Types of electromagnetic energy used in this category of alternative medicine include low-voltage electricity, radio waves and magnetic fields.

In contrast to proven types of electromagnetic energy that help to diagnose and treat disease — such as MRI, lasers, ionizing radiation and infrared rays — alternative electromagnetic therapies are not clinically proven to work against cancer or other diseases.

Although it is proven that electrical and magnetic energy exist in the human body, no studies have proven that electromagnetic therapy or any magnet have an effect on pain or any human ailment.

Chakra Balancing

Chakra balancing is a technique that aims to cleanse and balance the life-force energy in a person's body. Chakra balancing is offered by a variety of alternative energy healers, such as shamans or Reiki practitioners. Healers use several different methods to balance chakras. Some might involve the use of crystals, stones, essential oils and meditation. No clinical studies have been conducted on chakra balancing and little to no scientific research has investigated the theory of chakras.

The concept of chakras originated in India. Chakras are described as energy centers throughout the body that channel and store life-force energy. Approximately seven major chakras are defined, though some systems describe eight chakras and even microchakras within each energy center.

Anecdotal reports of chakra balancing say the therapy helps people to relax, reduce stress and increase well-being. Chakra balancing cannot treat or diagnose cancer. Like all complementary and alternative mesothelioma treatments, the therapy is meant to be a helpful addition to traditional cancer treatment, not a replacement for it.

Folk Medicines

Folk medicine has existed for as long as human beings have existed. In an effort to cope with an environment that was often dangerous, humans, and their ancestors, began to develop ways of lessening pain and treating physical and mental problems. At first, many of the ways of treating these problems undoubtedly came through trial and error, using various plants and other methods derived from observation of how animals reacted to and treated illnesses and injuries. Over time, individuals within family and tribal groups became more skilled at helping the sick and injured, and some of these became responsible for carrying out healing ceremonies, religious rituals, and other rites designed to ensure the safety and health of their communities.

Many of the methods for treating injuries and diseases have been passed down through families for generations, and some of these have been adopted for use by the medical profession. Those treatments not commonly believed to fit within the framework of modern medical practice are commonly identified as folk medicine. Illnesses whose etiologies are not recognized by Western medical practice are known as folk illnesses. Folk illnesses are shaped by the cultural and ethnic groups from which they emerge. They are specific to the cosmology of the cultural and ethnic group to which they belong and they have specific causative, diagnostic, preventative, and healing/curing practices that may vary significantly from how they may be viewed by modern medical practitioners. For example, liver grown is a folk illness found among Pennsylvania Germans. This illness is believed to occur when the liver has become attached to the ribs or some other part of the body cavity. The illness is thought to be more common among children and caused by exposure to a strong wind. It may also be the result of staying outside too long or from being shaken up while traveling. In the American South, the most common symptom in a child is failure to thrive in the child. The illness is diagnosed by feeling the lower chest and seeking to find the flesh pulled inward. Treatment may involve stretching the child's arms and legs behind them to loosen the liver or by passing them through a warm horse collar, bramble bush, or other similar process.

It is important to understand that some folk illnesses have common symptoms that are treated by Western medical practitioners, while other symptoms may not be understood by Western medicine to mean the same sort of thing. In the previous example, failure to thrive has a specific Western medical connotation and treatment approach that is different from that employed by those believing in liver grown.

In attempting to understand folk medicine, a number of researchers have noted that these remedies are often learned and passed down from parent to child, and the explanations for illness causation and treatment go hand in hand with this learning process. They have come to classify folk medicine into four major categories: the patient world, the natural world, the social world, and the supernatural world. The patient world is concerned with illnesses caused by factors that the patient has some control over, such as diet, smoking, drinking, and other lifestyle behaviors. The natural world includes problems related to animate and inanimate factors, including those caused by microorganisms and viruses; animal bites; and environmental factors such as pollution, pollens, poisons, and natural disasters. The social world covers interpersonal conflicts, including conditions caused by physical injury inflicted by one person on another, the stresses of daily living, and witchcraft and sorcery. The supernatural world includes illnesses caused by spirits, ancestors, or gods who have been offended through sinful behavior, the breaking of taboos, or other breaches of proper behavior.

Folk medicine practitioners use a variety of methods to treat illnesses. These practitioners go by many names, including shaman, curandero, root doctor, spirit medium, herbalist, native healer, medicine man, kahuna, and other related terms. Each has specific treatment approaches, which may include prayer, dancing, medicinal herbs, massage, sweat baths, coining (a process of rubbing the skin with a metal coin), cupping (a treatment used to draw blood to the surface of the skin by means of a small heated vessel made of horn, ceramic, or bamboo), hot and cold foods, and other practices not normally considered in modern biomedicine. Often these practitioners are the first to be consulted when a family member becomes ill. They are easy to access, tend to share the same illness causality beliefs, will come to the home day or night, and are much less expensive then a clinic, hospital, or doctor's office visit. Folk medicine practitioners are also often consulted when home remedies fail. If the practitioner also fails, then consultation with the biomedical community may occur.

In addition to the medical practices employed by traditional healers, there has also evolved a profusion of folk healing practices that are not seen by either the folk healer or modern health practitioner. These home healing practices are handed down by word of mouth and are used to treat a variety of illnesses, including anxiety and depression, coughs and colds, burns and sunburns, bladder and kidney infections, bedwetting, bites and stings, asthma, arthritis, birthing problems, bleeding, diarrhea, fever, infertility, insomnia, skin problems, and mouth and gum disorders. Almost every family has some specific home remedy that has been learned and passed down by older family members, and even in the face of more modern health beliefs they will continue to use these folk remedies before seeking other biomedical treatment methods. For instance, in many families an aloe leaf is used to treat a burn, rather than a burn ointment or spray from the pharmacy. Other examples of folk medical treatments include the use of American ginseng as a sedative or tonic in the Appalachian Mountains; celery seeds to help treat rheumatism among British and German immigrants to the United States; and ginger to treat gas or nausea in New England. In addition to these historical practices, the spectrum of folk medicine in the United States has been extended by the influx of new immigrant groups.

Magic animals have also been used in folk medical practices. Animal parts and by-products are used to treat certain illnesses or conditions—bird nests are used to prevent headaches, the tooth of a mole may be worn around the neck to prevent toothache, and fresh muskrat skin is used to prevent colds. Other animals thought to have healing properties include toads, snakes, eels, and earthworms.

Prayers are also used in folk medicine. In Appalachian and southern culture, "fire doctors" use prayer to alleviate the pain of burns. In Native-American and Asian cultures, prayer is used to cure soul-loss or ghost sickness. Prayer has been scientifically studied to determine its effects in helping people to get well or to feel better, and there is some evidence that it does have value in the treatment of illness and disease.

Other folk medicine remedies have been shown to be effective. One such remedy is the eating of live-culture yogurt to reduce vaginal yeast infections.

The placebo effect can, however, play a part in the efficacy of a treatment. A strong belief in a certain treatment can yield a positive outcome, even with a treatment that has been shown scientifically not to work. At the same time, some folk remedies, like modern medicines, can have serious, and sometimes fatal, side effects. Plants gathered to treat an illness may have been prepared improperly, or the wrong plant may have been picked along with the correct one, tainting the remedy. Some preparations may be too strong for some patients, particularly infants or those weakened by serious illness. The use of any herbal preparation should therefore be approached with great caution, even if purchased at a health-food store or other commercial outlet. Herbal remedies are not well regulated and may be dangerous to take.

Folk medicine exists side by side with modern medical practices, and is often at odds with it. This is primarily because it very often does not conform with what is scientifically known about the causes of illness and disease and what are thought to be the most effective medical treatments. For those who use and believe in folk medical practices, their knowledge has been acquired from generations of others that have used the treatments. Folk medicine traditions stress the importance of balance and harmony within the body. A sense that each person is connected to the earth and the cosmos is very important, as is the belief that an illness should be treated with every resource available. Herbal preparations, prayer, magic, diet, exercise, and proper social relations are all viable tools in the effort to maintain health. For public health practitioners, an awareness of the diversity of health beliefs and practices that may be encountered among those who use more traditional folk medicine approaches, and the ability to suspend judgement about those who use them, is an important step in learning to work more effectively with the diverse folk medicine traditions they encounter in their practice.

Magnet Therapy

Magnetic field therapy uses different kinds of magnets on the body to help boost your overall health. It may also help treat certain conditions.

There are several types, including:

- Static magnetic field therapy: In this, you touch a magnet to your skin somehow. You might wear a magnetic bracelet or other magnetized jewelry. It could be a bandage with a magnet in it, or you may wear a magnet as a shoe insole. You could also sleep on a special mattress pad with a magnet in it.
- Electrically charged magnetic therapy (electromagnetic therapy): The magnets

you use here have an electric charge. Treatment with electromagnetic therapy usually comes through an electric pulse.

- Magnetic therapy with acupuncture: Magnets go on the same sections of your skin that an acupuncturist would probably focus on in an acupuncture session. You may hear these areas called your energy pathways or channels.

How it Works

Your body naturally has magnetic and electric fields. All your molecules have a small amount of magnetic energy in them. The thought behind magnetic field therapy is that certain problems happen because your magnetic fields are out of balance. If you put a magnetic field near your body, it's believed things will go back to normal.

Ions like calcium and potassium help your cells send signals. In tests, scientists have seen magnets change how these ions act. However, so far, there isn't evidence that magnets have the same effect on cells when they're in your body.

What it's used for

Most magnetic field therapy is a treatment option for different types of pain, like in your feet and back.

Scientists have specifically studied its use for:

- Arthritis pain,
- Wound healing,
- Insomnia,
- Headaches,
- Fibromyalgia pain.

Not Adviced for

While it's generally safe for most people to wear low-intensity static magnets, it's not a good idea to have magnetic field therapy if you:

- Use a pacemaker,
- Have an insulin pump,
- Are pregnant.

You should also take off any magnets before having an X-ray or getting an MRI.

Some people who have magnetic field therapy have side effects like:

- Pain,
- Nausea,
- Dizziness.

However, these side effects are rare.

Massage Therapy

Massage therapy has a long history in cultures around the world. Today, people use many different types of massage therapy for a variety of health-related purposes. In the United States, massage therapy is often considered part of complementary and alternative medicine (CAM), although it does have some conventional uses.

- Scientific evidence on massage therapy is limited. Scientists are not yet certain what changes occur in the body during massage, whether they influence health, and, if so, how. The National Center for Complementary and Alternative Medicine (NCCAM) is sponsoring studies to answer these questions and identify the purposes for which massage may be most helpful.
- Massage therapy appears to have few serious risks if it is used appropriately and provided by a trained massage professional.

Massage therapy dates back thousands of years. References to massage appear in writings from ancient China, Japan, India, Arabic nations, Egypt, Greece (Hippocrates defined medicine as "the art of rubbing"), and Rome.

Massage became widely used in Europe during the Renaissance. In the 1850s, two American physicians who had studied in Sweden introduced massage therapy in the United States, where it became popular and was promoted for a variety of health purposes. With scientific and technological advances in medical treatment during the 1930s and 1940s, massage fell out of favor in the United States. Interest in massage revived in the 1970s, especially among athletes.

What are the Health Benefits of Massage Therapy?

According to the 2007 National Health Interview Survey, which included a comprehensive survey of CAM use by Americans, an estimated 18 million U.S. adults and 700,000 children had received massage therapy in the previous year.

People use massage for a variety of health-related purposes, including to relieve pain, rehabilitate sports injuries, reduce stress, increase relaxation, address anxiety and depression, and aid general wellness.

Massage Therapy

The term "massage therapy" encompasses many different techniques. In general, therapists press, rub, and otherwise manipulate the muscles and other soft tissues of the body. They most often use their hands and fingers, but may use their forearms, elbows, or feet.

Types of Massage Therapy

In Swedish massage, the therapist uses long strokes, kneading, deep circular movements, vibration, and tapping. Sports massage is similar to Swedish massage, adapted specifically to the needs of athletes. Among the many other examples are deep tissue massage and trigger point massage, which focuses on myofascial trigger points -- muscle "knots" that are painful when pressed and can cause symptoms elsewhere in the body.

What do Massage Therapists do in Treating Patients?

Massage therapists work in a variety of settings, including private offices, hospitals, nursing homes, studios, and sport and fitness facilities. Some also travel to patients' homes or workplaces. They usually try to provide a calm, soothing environment.

Therapists usually ask new patients about symptoms, medical history, and desired results. They may also perform an evaluation through touch, to locate painful or tense areas and determine how much pressure to apply.

Typically, the patient lies on a table, either in loose-fitting clothing or undressed (covered with a sheet, except for the area being massaged). The therapist may use oil or lotion to reduce friction on the skin. Sometimes, people receive massage therapy while sitting in a chair. A massage session may be fairly brief, but may also last an hour or even longer.

How does Massage Therapy Affect the Body?

Although scientific research on massage therapy - whether it works and, if so, how - is limited, there is evidence that massage may benefit some patients. Conclusions generally cannot yet be drawn about its effectiveness for specific health conditions.

According to one analysis, however, research supports the general conclusion that massage therapy is effective. The studies included in the analysis suggest that a single session of massage therapy can reduce "state anxiety" (a reaction to a particular situation), blood pressure, and heart rate, and multiple sessions can reduce "trait anxiety" (general anxiety-proneness), depression, and pain. In addition, recent studies suggest that massage may benefit certain conditions, for example:

- A 2008 review of 13 clinical trials found evidence that massage might be useful for chronic low-back pain. Clinical practice guidelines issued in 2007 by the American Pain Society and the American College of Physicians recommend that physicians consider using certain CAM therapies, including massage (as well as acupuncture, chiropractic, progressive relaxation, and yoga), when patients with chronic low-back pain do not respond to conventional treatment.
- A multisite study of more than 300 hospice patients with advanced cancer concluded that massage may help to relieve pain and improve mood for these patients.
- A study of 64 patients with chronic neck pain found that therapeutic massage was more beneficial than a self-care book, in terms of improving function and relieving symptoms.

There are numerous theories about how massage therapy may affect the body. For example, the "gate control theory" suggests that massage may provide stimulation that helps to block pain signals sent to the brain. Other theories suggest that massage might stimulate the release of certain chemicals in the body, such as serotonin or endorphins, or cause beneficial mechanical changes in the body. However, additional studies are needed to test the various theories.

What are Side Effects and Risks of Massage Therapy?

Massage therapy appears to have few serious risks - if it is performed by a properly trained therapist and if appropriate cautions are followed. The number of serious injuries reported is very small. Side effects of massage therapy may include temporary pain or discomfort, bruising, swelling, and a sensitivity or allergy to massage oils.

Cautions about massage therapy include the following:

- Vigorous massage should be avoided by people with bleeding disorders or low blood platelet counts, and by people taking blood-thinning medications such as warfarin.
- Massage should not be done in any area of the body with blood clots, fractures, open or healing wounds, skin infections, or weakened bones (such as from osteoporosis or cancer), or where there has been a recent surgery.
- Although massage therapy appears to be generally safe for cancer patients, they should consult their oncologist before having a massage that involves deep or

intense pressure. Any direct pressure over a tumor usually is discouraged. Cancer patients should discuss any concerns about massage therapy with their oncologist.

- Pregnant women should consult their health care provider before using massage therapy.

Reflexology

Reflexology is a systematic practice in which applying some pressure to any particular points on the feet and hands give impacts on the health of related parts of the body. Each point of the pressure acts as the sensors on the feet and hands and is links with different parts of body specifically. These sensors will be stimulated by applying the reflexology technique in order to improve the blood and energy circulation, give sense of relaxation, and maintain the homoeostasis. Reflexology session can be improved by other elements such as aromatherapy, peaceful music, and good environment settings. There is a term in reflexology called reflex zone therapy. Reflex zone therapy is where the body is divided into ten longitudinal zones from head to toe. In the reflex zone therapy, there are five zones on both sides of the body in which each zone diverge down the particular arm, and also continue straight down the body and down the particular leg to line up with a toe on the respective foot. Practitioners usually choose the suitable technique to be applied to the reflex zone therapy to gain optimized efficiency and impact. Reflexology is a complementary therapy instead of an alternative therapy to other treatments which patient already has based on reflexology maps. Complementary therapies nowadays are applied in many of palliative care or to alleviate a problem without dealing with the underlying cause in order to make patient's emotional, physiological, and spiritual health improve and increase the value of their life. Two methods of reflexology that have been accepted internationally are Ingham method and Rwo Shur method. The first method does not use any tools in its practice and the second method utilizes the use of tools such as a wooden stick. There are five theories that support how reflexology gives impacts to body health. First and second basic theories are related to energy. Energy theory advocates that body parts can communicate using electromagnetic fields and the communication can be blocked based on the surrounding respectively. Third and fourth theories indicate that energy flow can be restored and the fourth is about the pathway which is blocked can be opened. The last theory proposes that reflexology can break up the lactic acid crystal that usually deposited in the feet and allow energy to flow efficiently.

Modern reflexology technique has been used since 60 years ago and now more scientific and clinical research have been conducted because of their positive effects in reducing and alleviating the symptoms associated with certain diseases. Reflexology gives benefits to certain groups of people and generally does not cause any harmful effects as long as certain precautions are taken by the patients with certain medical circumstances. Each person has a different body system condition, so results from reflexology treatment could differ from one person to another. Based on latest research conducted, reflexology seems to be effective in helping the body systems to return to its natural state. One of the most significant current discussions in reflexology is its effectiveness in tackling several symptoms of diseases. The level of disease conditions and pain are reduced as the patients receive reflexology treatment. It has been suggested by a Swiss study that patients who have undergone reflexology sessions showed a significant decrease in the amount of medication needed. As a complementary therapy, reflexology seems to work better with conventional treatment to treat certain diseases. The most significant current discussions in reflexology practice are related to the aspect of health, safety, and hygiene. Other than that, the principles and practice of reflexology as a complementary therapy is important to make sure the application of this therapy is reliable.

Benefits of Reflexology

Reflexology has been chosen by most people to treat their body health problems because it offers high level of safety and effectiveness. It also offers natural treatment without consuming drugs and it is easy to use. Learning reflexology and its application is quite easy, there is no limitation for people to apply it anytime and anywhere. Its effectiveness in treating the root of some diseases may lead to many benefits in health concern such as it helps in easing day-to-day stresses and alleviates the effects from injury and illness. However, it is not used in diagnosing processes.

Stress contributes up to 80% for the development of any illness. Other 20% of stress will influence other conditions. Reflexology offers common benefits and one of themis reducing stress by applying pressure to the specific area at feet and hands which may induce general relaxation while relaxing the targeted area concurrently. Reflexology is one of the ways to interrupt the pattern of repetitive stress that people usually have according to their lifestyle. They will operate more effective with a number of reflexology sessions because the first application will intervene the stress operation and further sessions will improve the body condition. Besides, reflexology also allows the body to get off fromany stress in everyday life.

Pain is a stressor in the body system and any injury occurs to any part of the body will cause the whole system to be stressed. Endorphin is a body's natural pain-relieving chemical will be released as a response to reflexology. Endorphin teaches the body how to adapt any injuries. Those who practice reflexology in their life believe that healing from any injuries comes from the role of reflexology.

It generally improves body health condition and well-being in terms of physical, emotional, and spiritual level. In simple sentence, people choose reflexology because:

- The treatment is free from any drugs and chemical, and it is a wide option for many health problems.

- Its ability to reduce pain.
- It helps body to maintain the dexterity and locomotion ability.
- It promotes general sense of relaxation especially overused or tired hands, feet, and the whole body parts.
- It stimulates the release of body's pain-relieving chemicals.
- As a prevention from any illness.
- It promotes recovery process from any injury particularly at any region at hands and feet.

Maps of Reflexology

Different maps representing the body reflex areas on the palms and feet are presented in this topic.

A series of banded reflex area on the top of the left hand represents the left hand side of the body from the top left side of the head to the knee. Specifically, reflex area for lymph glands, groin, and fallopian tubes encircled the wrist.

This reflex area represents the right side of the body. There is an invisible point at the base of the hand's long bones which is called as waistline. This line divided the hand into two parts. The upper back reflex area lies on the above of the line whereas lower back, hips, and internal organs located below it.

This reflex area is related to the left side of the body. Reflex area of the spine lies inside whereas the shoulders are positioned outside. The head and neck reflex area are located on the fingers with the tailbone near the wrist.

Two sides of the body have different internal organs. This makes each reflex area is specifically for certain organs. This reflex area represents the right side of the body. For example, the reflex area for liver is only available on the right side of the palm.

The reflex area of spine lies on the inside part of the top left foot whereas shoulders on the outside. Lung, chest, breast, and upper back assemble in one reflex area.

This reflex area relates to the right side of the body including arm and leg. There is awaistline at the point halfway down each foot. The upper back and all organs related to it are positioned above this line whereas lower back and internal organs are located below the line. The lymph gland and groin reflex wrap around the ankle.

This map represents the reflex area of the right side of the body. For example, shoulder reflex area relates to the right shoulder. Liver reflex area is much larger on the right side compared to the left side due to the position of the liver itself which is mostly on the right side of the body.

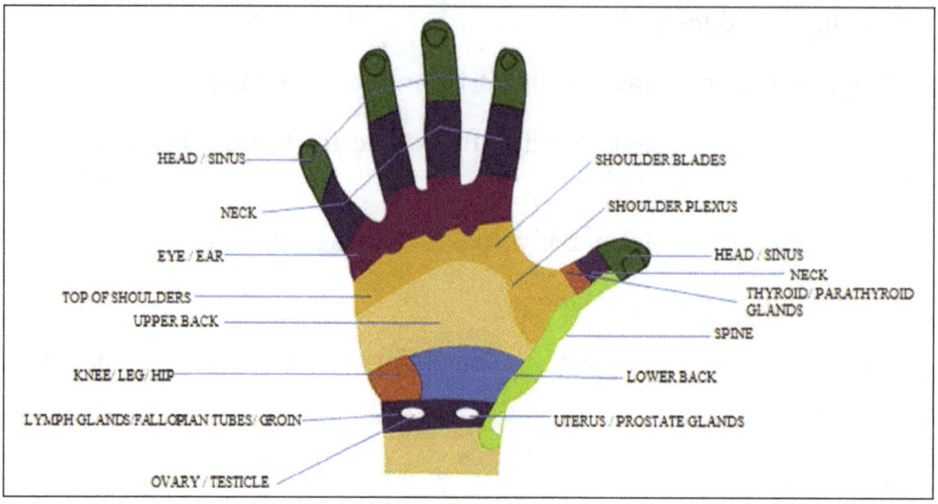

Top of left hand.

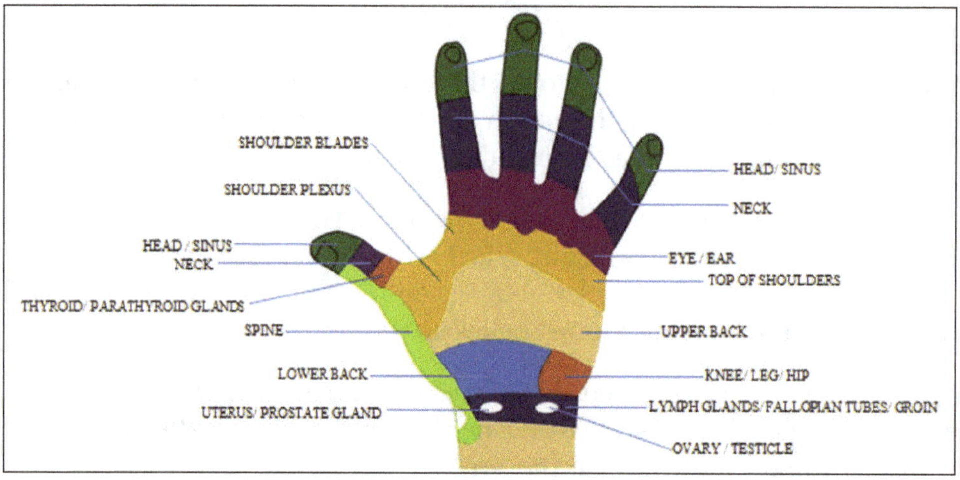

Top of right hand.

It represents the reflex area of the left side of the body with certain organs involved. The reflex area of heart, stomach, and pancreas are larger on the left sole compared to the right sole because these organs are generally located on the left side of the body.

Reflex Zone Therapy

Reflex zone is the region in the zone therapy that illustrates its interconnection with the whole parts of the body. Pressure applied to this region will help specific organ or particular part to alleviate the pain and symptoms of a disease. According to the theory, there is an invisible pathway that runs along the body in a vertical form based on the lines instead of reflexology maps in which each point on the soles of hand and feet correspond to a specific organ. Reflex zone therapy represents five zones in both sides of the feet. This zone is running along the whole body parts from top of the head until the tips of the toes and fingers and the whole body is divided into ten reflex zones. Each zone interconnects with different parts of the body. Reflex zone therapy-specific organ relationship is presented.

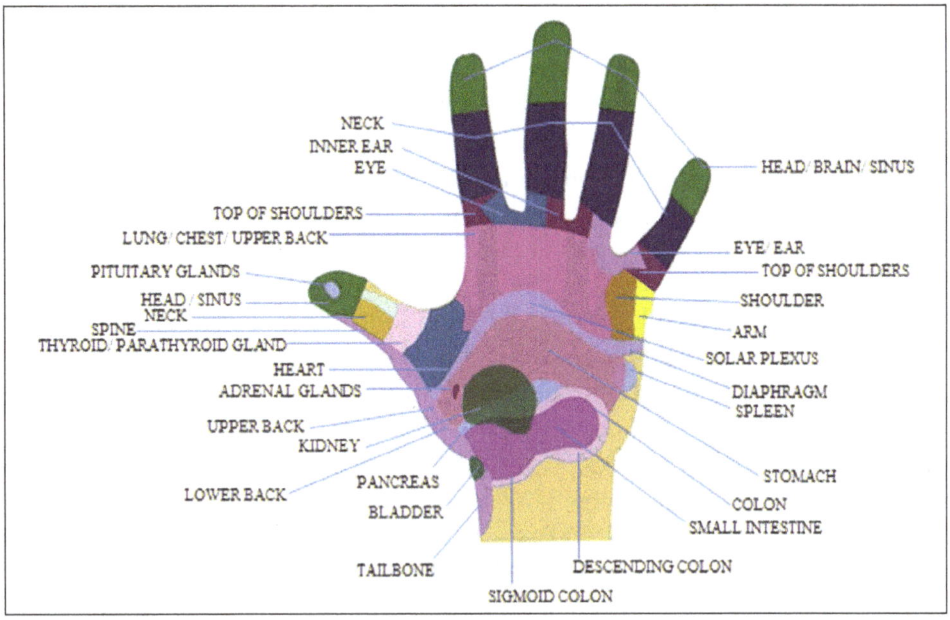

Left palm.

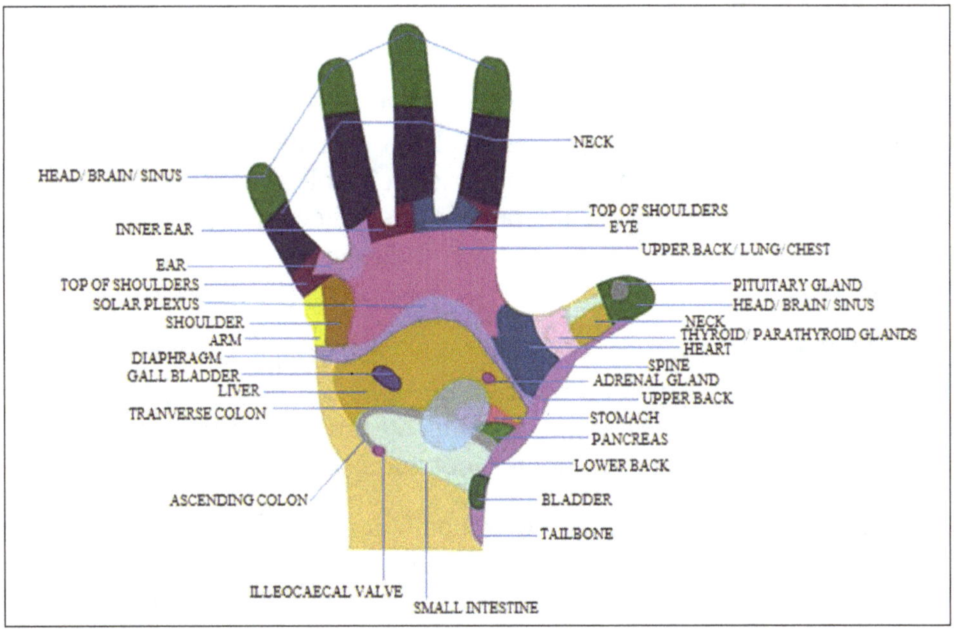

Right palm.

Different Applications of Reflexology and the Effects of Reflexology

The findings by a recent study have confirmed the efficacy of reflexology by recording 31% of pain reduction among the patients with back pain. Quinn et al. reported that the pain intensity score decreased to an average extent in the experimental group. Poole et al. demonstrated that there was a significant difference between the control and experimental groups before and after the reflexology treatment.

A statistic has showed that there are more than 5000 registered reflexology centres in Malaysia. Currently, reflexology is a big industry in Malaysia with a huge unexploited potential for tourism and human capital, especially for disabled people. Owing to that, Ministry of Health has published the good practice guidelines for reflexology in 2011 to strengthen and govern its operations. Different use of reflexology and the effect of reflexology are listed below:

1. Low back pain management: A study by an author found that patients who suffered from low back pain usually show good effect in terms of their pain management when they have reflexology as the complementary treatment. In this study, the author used VAS scores to indicate the level of pain of the patient. The author added that this complementary treatment can be used as one of the treatment to reduce low back pain but further study on it must be conducted.

2. Migraine/headache: Patients were referred to a physiotherapist for the six months and the effect of the therapy was recorded by several methods such as qualitative interviews, headache diaries, and questionnaire. The results came out with 55% of them experienced relief, 23% expressed no further recurrence of symptoms, and the rest 11% stopped taking their medications.

3. Stroke: Stroke is the condition where the blood supply to the brain is interrupted because of some reasons that may cause many health problems. It usually occurs due to blood vessels ruptures. Many patients have tried reflexology as the alternative therapy in order to recover from strokes. The practitioners believe that pressure that they exerted on a particular point on reflex areas may induce a positive outcome and physical changes to the body.

4. Stress reduction: In 2000, Hayes and Cox published a paper in which they described that there are significant reduction in stress in which can be determine by measuring the heart rate, respirations, and mean atrial blood pressure of the patients who have about two to three sessions of five minutes foot massage.

5. Multiple sclerosis: An author found that a patient who afflict multiple sclerosis and choose reflexology as the complementary treatment for a period of time had notable symptom relief. It is measured by considering urinary symptoms, parenthesis, spasticity, and muscle strength as the parameters. All parameters showed a remarkable improvement except for muscle strength.

6. Peripheral neuropathy in diabetes mellitus: Previous research has showed that reflexology can reduce the peripheral neuropathy of a patient who suffers from type 2 diabetes mellitus. 76 patients ranged from 40-79 years old were listed from public health

centres in Busan City. Tactile response to monofilament and intensity of the symptoms of peripheral neuropathy were used as the variable outcomes in this study. Tingling sensation and pain were reduced and tactile was more sensitive to 10 g force monofilament. The author added that the reflexology can be used as one of the interventions for encouraging foot care in patients who have diabetes mellitus. It also can be measured based on glycaemic control and nerve conductivity which show improvement with reflexology.

7. Asthma: 20 asthmatic patients were chosen to be the subject for active treatment and another 20 patients were chosen to have reflexology session. According to a recent research conducted by the author, there are no significant differences between the groups having active session and placebo session of reflexology. However, when the analysis of the symptoms diaries was carried out, the results showed that there were significant differences between both groups especially when it was conducted together with subconscious unblinding pattern of study.

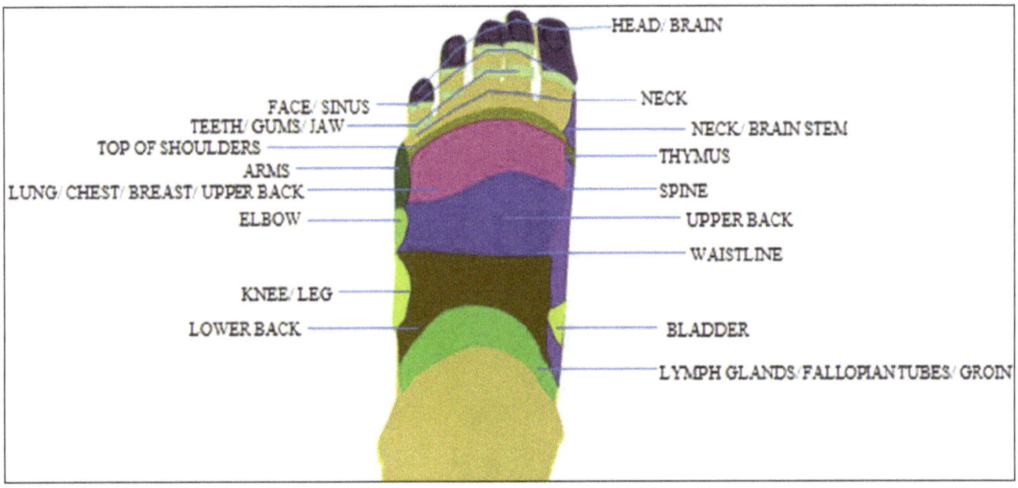

Top of left foot.

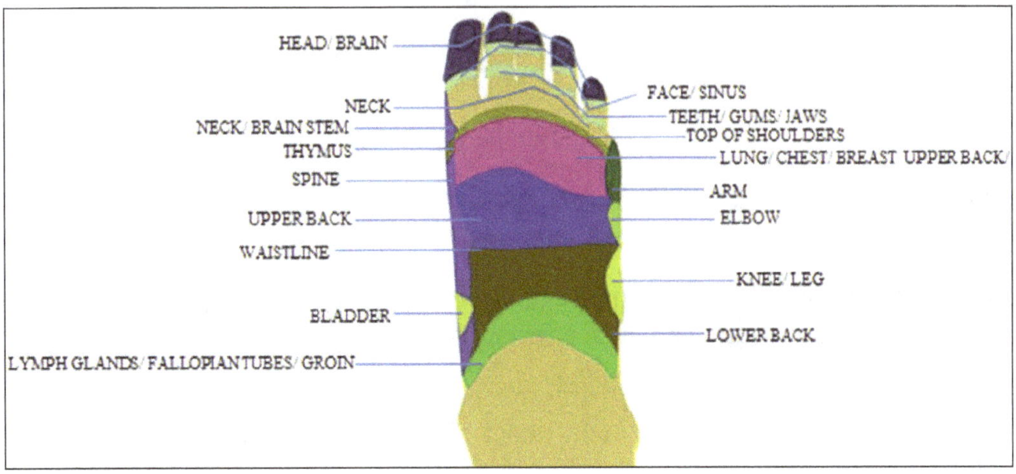

Top of right foot.

Evidence-based Practice

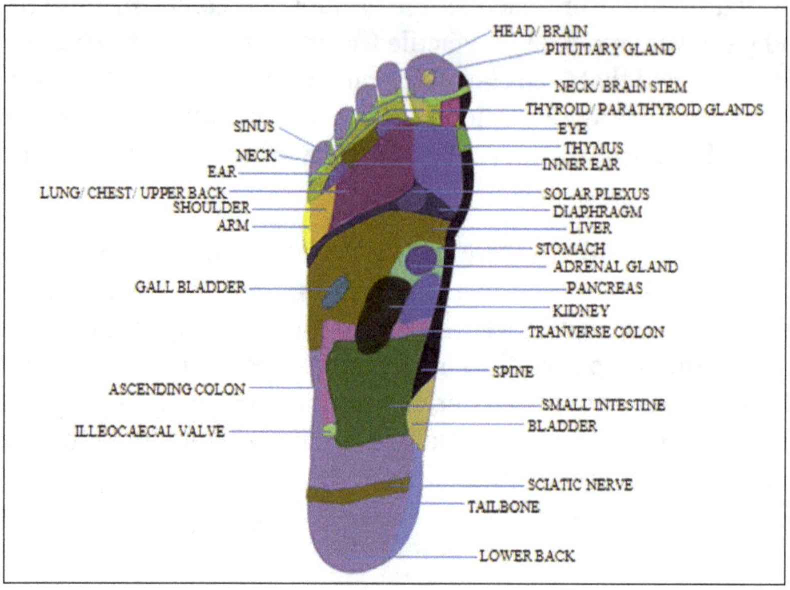

Right sole.

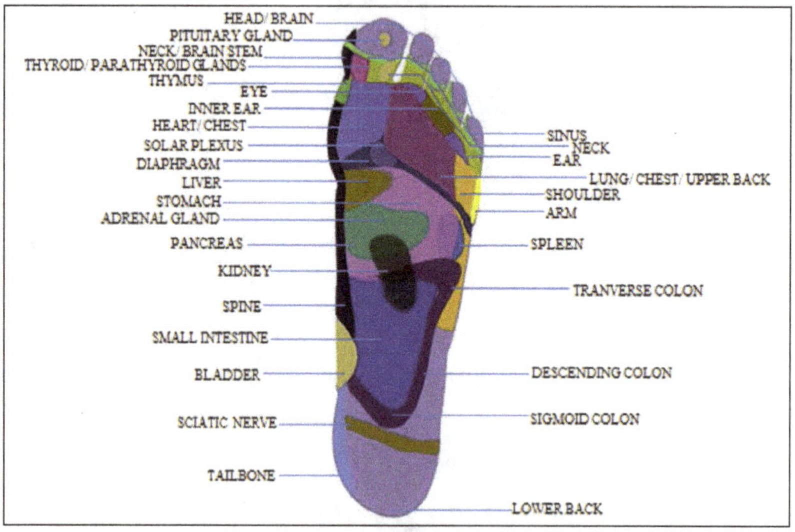

Left sole.

From ten systematic reviews, it is safe to conclude that until now reflexology does not have sufficient evidence to support its clinical use.

There are also many conditions of patients where we need to avoid applying reflexology because it will give unwanted adverse effects.

1. Pregnancy but only for the first trimester period: Practitioners may be accused to have caused the case if there is unlucky miscarriage after the therapy. So practitioners must take the precaution steps by avoiding patients in their first trimester of pregnancy.

2. Diarrhoea and vomiting: Reflexology may cause overstimulation of the body system and may exasperate the condition of the infections.

3. Localized skin disease at hand, feet, and ears: Hand, feet, and ears are the area of reflexology. If there are infections on this area, reflexology can be hurtful and exasperate the existence conditions.

4. Localized inflammation or swelling of the feet, hand, and ears: Similar situation will happen as the skin diseases worsen due to the practitioner's hand or finger motion on the area of therapy.

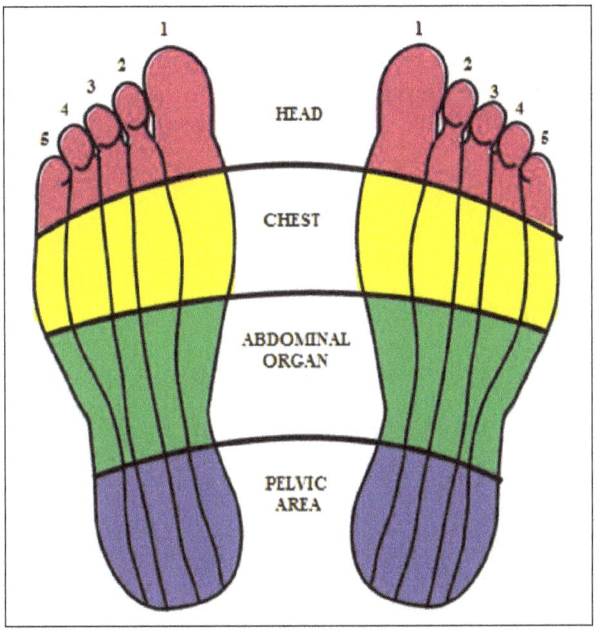

Zone therapy reflex.

5. Fever and any infectious diseases whether systemic or localized: In order to fight the infection, the body system which is already stressed will be over stimulated in the patient who suffers from any infections and at the same time having this therapy.

6. Continuing extreme negative reaction to reflexology: If the patient feels uncomfortable and their body health continuously worsens after having this therapy, it is advisable to reconsider the suitability of reflexology for the client.

Shiatsu

Shiatsu is an ancient non-invasive therapeutic technique, a comprehensive treatment system based on the same concepts and roots with Chinese Acupuncture and Traditional Chinese Medicine (TCM).

According to this theory, the human body and its internal organs function with the power and influence of Chi Energy.

The imbalance between our mental, physical, emotional and spiritual world, is the reason that our body gets sick. What Shiatsu does is, to restore this balance of energy in the body and bring a harmony between these aspects of our life.

Shiatsu is performed by finger pressure (instead of needles) on the acupoints.

Shiatsu was developed in Japan by combining a Chinese type of massage, the Anma and Western physical therapy techniques.

The Shiatsu techniques include stretching, grip and inclination of therapist's body weight over many parts of the recipient's body.

The objective is to improve:

- The energy flow,
- The blood circulation,
- The flexibility and,
- The Posture of the body Pressure and contact is applied through,
- Hands,
- Thumbs,
- Fingers,
- Forearms,
- knees and,
- Feet.

It is performed with the recipient in various positions such as supine, side, prone, sitting. The treatment focuses mainly along specific channels ("Meridians") from where the body Chi energy passes through.

Although Shiatsu literally means 'finger pressure', the soul of Shiatsu is communication through touch. Shiatsu which meets the needs of the recipient cannot be achieved only with technical skills and intellectual study. So that it will be effective, requires sensitivity so that we feel and influence positively the quality of energy that exists within the recipient's body.

Shiatsu for Common Ailments

Shiatsu cannot be used for treating diseases, as for such cases we must reach out to our doctor.

However, what it can offer is:

- To relieve from some symptoms,
- To prevent and minimize some undesired evolution and,
- To complement the treatment of some specific health,
- professionals (if permitted),,
- Usually, some of such discomfort cases are,
- Mental and Physical fatigue,
- Stress,
- Worry,
- Insomnia,
- Back pain and sciatica,
- Period pains.

Performing Shiatsu

Shiatsu is done with the recipient wearing light and comfortable cotton clothes, usually lying on a comfortable cotton or futon mattress on the floor. Usually, an experienced therapist will use some pillows under the recipient's feet or hands, to cover the gap and absorb any possible mechanical restoration and traction during the pressure.

The position can be supine, prone, lateral or sitting.

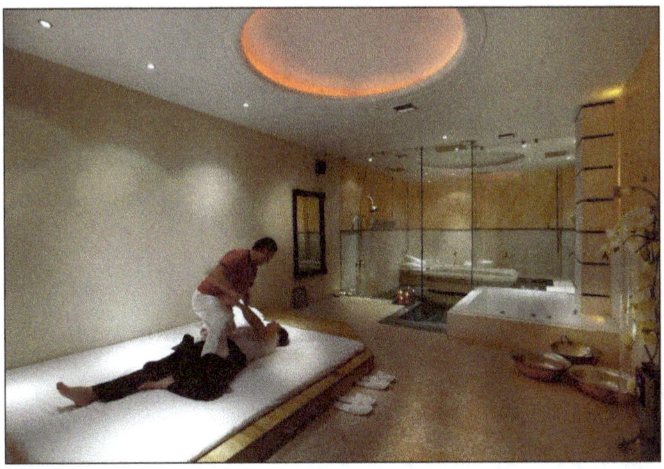

There is continuous contact between the recipient and the Shiatsu therapist, while the first relaxes and the second maintains continuous physical, energy, and emotional communication in a relaxed meditative atmosphere. Do not forget that this is an energy healing technique.

Thumbs, elbows, fingers, forearms, feet pressure is used by the therapist. Also, some stretches from the Western Physio or Oriental Yoga.

The fact that there is no need for the recipient to take off his/ her clothes, like they do in a Deep Tissue massage, Shiatsu is suitable in any place or in any time of the day.

Provided there is appropriate peaceful atmosphere without noises that distract our attention. No special equipment is required such as massage oils, only the expert hands of the therapist.

When is Not Suitable to Do Shiatsu?

Generally Shiatsu is a very safe technique. Here it holds the same with the other massage treatments. However, we would avoid just to press on some points or localy on some specific areas. Such points are, four points which may cause miscarriage to a pregnant woman or undesired premature birth and some points contraindicated in some people with hypertension or hypotension. Also, we never press points with inflammation, edema, trauma, varicose veins or pimples.

An experienced professional therapist will first take a short medical history from the client and then will go through the Shiatsu session.

Traditional Chinese Medicine – Some Basic Terms

One to understand how Shiatsu works, first should consider the core of Traditional Chinese Medicine (TCM), in other words how this ancient Chinese system treats the disease. In Western Medicine, a doctor will deal more with the effects of the disease and will try to minimize or eliminate them completely.

In TCM, the therapist will make a completely different diagnosis. He/she will observe the whole picture of the patient, the overall external appearance, the way the patient moves, speaks and behaves, until the color of the patient's urine, the tastes that prefers and his/her emotional state. The therapist will try to build a profile of the patient, which will consist of some "Syndromes disharmony."

The Oriental therapist, the Acupuncturist or the Shiatsu therapist is expected to treat this Disharmony and to restore it to its original equilibrium (state).

The Energy Chi Concept

Chi is the vital force that supports every activity of the human body, mind and spirit. According to the Chinese theory of Taoism, Chi is everywhere in the universe surrounding us. It is in the air we breathe, the food we eat, inside us as a legacy of our parents.

The Chinese character for Chi suggests that it is something which, at the same time is material and intangible:

Steam, gas # (uncooked) rice = Chi

This clearly shows that Chi can be as intangible as steam and so dense material as rice. It also shows that, Chi is a thin element (steam) coming from something concentrated (rice), such as steam produced when the rice is cooked.

Chi has been translated like many concepts, such are: Energy, Material Force, Matter, Ether, Material Energy, Life Force, Vital Force, Vital Dynamic, and Moving Energy.

The inability to be translated exactly stems from its nature of taking various forms of expression. Chi nourishes the vital organs of the human body, the Blood and other Body Fluids and our Mind. In Traditional Chinese Medicine bibliography you will see the word blood written with a capital B. This is to distinguish the difference between the red fluid of blood that runs in our veins from the Blood, one of the shapes Chi gets and one of the Vital Forces.

It is also responsible for all the processes of life, from conception, childbirth, to growth and death.

'Chi produces the human body, exactly like the water becomes ice. As the water freezes (and becomes ice) so Chi coagulates to form the human body. When the ice melts is water. When a person dies, becomes spirit (Shen) again. It is called spirit, just like molten ice is changing its name to water.

The Elements Yin and Yang

It is the oldest (700 BC) and significant philosophical theory in Chinese medicine, which is completely different from any Western. Therefore, according to this theory, everything in life, every phenomenon can be exactly what it is, and also it's opposite. Also, the Yin element contains within it the seed of Yang and the Yang Element contains within it the seed of Yin Element.

Each element complements and supports each other. They are two phases in a circular motion. For example, the day alternates to night progressively, there is time of day that contains little dark and there is time of night that contains light in it. Like the Five Elements, so Yin-Yang have some specific characteristics, qualities, properties. Some of them are Light-Dark, Motion-Rest, Material and Intangible, Energy- Matter, Water-Fire, etc.

Yin-Yang keeps under its power and controls some internal organs. Between them there are some principles of co-existence and relationship, which when they are violated a disharmony and imbalance is occurred to human organs and body.

The Five Elements

This is an ancient Theory (1000 -770 BC), that together with the Yin-Yang theory they are the basis of Traditional Chinese Medicine. The term has been used by ancient Greek philosophers, Air-Fire-Earth-Water, roots, elements, primordial bodies, etc. In fact, it is about five processes, five qualities; five stages of a cycle or alternating phenomena. The 5 Elements are Wood, Fire, Earth, Metal and Water.

The Five Elements

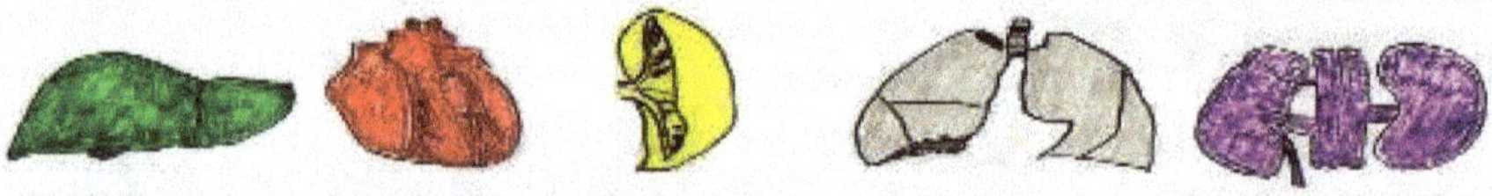

LIVER	HEART	SPLEEN	LUNGS	KIDNEYS
Wood	Fire	Earth	Metal	Water
Spring	Summer	Late Summer	Autumn	Winter
Gallbladder	Small Intestine	Stomach	Large Intestine	Urinary Bladder
Wind	Heat	Damp	Dry	Cold
Green	Red	Yellow	White	Black

Each element has specific characteristics, qualities, properties that in Shiatsu practice are used in Physiology, in Pathology, in the diagnosis and recovery strategy that we will pursue.

Some of these are the flavors, sounds, odors, some senses, climates, etc. Each item is under the influence of an internal vital organ such as the Liver, Heart, Spleen, Large Intestine, Kidney, Gall Blader, etc. Each organ influences, governs, controls, affects another and is controlled and affected by someone else. There is a regular balanced cycle of control of all previous procedures, but there is also an imbalanced cycle and one insulting cycle.

As is mentioned above, the therapist who uses T.C.M, the Acupuncturist or the Shiatsu therapist is called to restore this Disharmony and to restore it to its original equilibrium (state).

The Meridians-What is Tsubo?

According to Chinese Medicine, energy is released in some channels on the surface of our body. The Meridians are the pathways for the circulation of Chi and present in everyone's body. Meridians have been identified and every one of them takes its name from the specified internal organ passes through or is connected eg Heart Meridian, Stomach Meridian, Bladder Channel, etc.

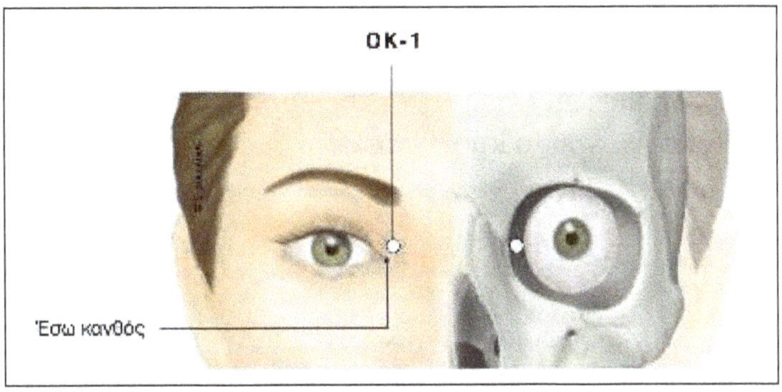

Over the Channels there are specific points, on which the Shiatsu practioners puts pressure or the acupuncturist's needles. The points are numerous and located on or near veins, arteries, tendons, nerves. And no, I am afraid they are not the points of the lymphatic system, as some health professional's claim, rationalizing the system of Traditional Chinese Medicine with Western mindset of conventional medicine.

The points in Japanese are called Tsubo and these in turn have names. In Chinese, for some of the points are used somewhat poetic names such as "Gate of Life/Mingmen", for some others quite illustrative names as "Intersection of 3 Yin / Sanyinjiao". In English we use the name of the Channel belonging point numbered, such as Du -4 and Spleen-6 respectively for the previous two.

Each point has specific functions, techniques by which is pressed, actions that it does, and sometimes contraindications. So, one point can strengthen an internal organ or Yin or Yang and other point can calm or descent the Chi. Some enhance the (birth) delivery, so if you do not want to have unexpected results, do not press it! A well, efficiently and professionally educated therapist of Shiatsu, in order to identify the points should certainly have learned first Anatomy, Physiology and Pathology and point location.

The Kyo/Jitsu Concept

In the system of Zen Shiatsu, whose founder was the Japanese teacher of Shiatsu Shizuto Masunaga (1925-1981), there are the concepts Kyo / Jitsu. They have been translated as Empty / Full, ie deficient and excess Chi respectively, referring to a tsubo point.

The Jitsu/Full points are easily identifiable by touch (and by the kin eye sometimes), as they would usually are protruding and aching, eg in a back. The Kyo / Empty points are identified with difficulty and usually they are deeper in the body. The Shiatsu therapist should have enough experience to distinguish the difference, and to turn them into their original balance effectively. This is the difference of a good shiatsu session with a very good session Shiatsu.

The teacher of Zen Shiatsu, Chris Jarmey whose courses I had the fortune and honor to attend many times, in his book – 'Shiatsu, The complete guide' (with G. Mojey and my greek teacher Ilaira Bouratinou) likens the Kyo/Jitsu like a house which someone is banging the door. Depending ie, if someone is inside the house and not or someone can be inside but does not wishes any visitors or the opposite, someone welcomes you and shows you he was expecting you to knock the door.

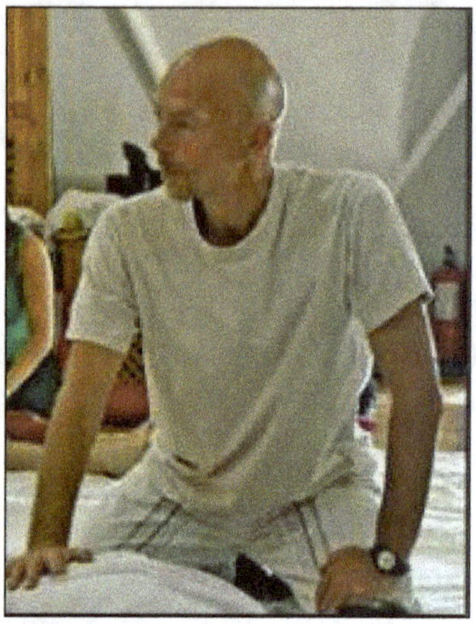

The Vital Substances Concept

As Vital substances in TCM is meant Qi, Blood, the Essence and the Body Fluids. That is, another powerful system of important functions. About Chi we discussed above. What we have not said is that Chi protects, nourishes, warms our bodies, transforms and transports food and our blood, and also holds and uplifts. With the term Blood (with a capital A) we do are not just referring to our blood, but a form of Chi, more dense and material (ie Yin). Blood is the "Mother of Chi, it nourishes the body and the mind and cools down the internal organs.The deficiency of blood cause imbalances mainly in Mind.

'Jing' Essence is a fine term of TCM, which one cannot find an equal term in Western Medicine and it's meaning is hard to explain.

The human body takes energy from the air we breathe, the food we eat and from a third source, the Essence. What we mean by Essence is, imagine a substance which exists within us inherited from our parents! This substance that nourishes the fetus inherited from our parents at conception. It affects our development, our reproduction and sexual maturation, and in general what we call our "constitution" among some other things. It's what makes each of us unique.

The Essence is unique and is replenished very to not at all. According to some specialists Yoga, Tai Chi/Qi Gong, Asian Martial arts, etc. help to be replenished. Imagine it as some money left for you by your parents to a Bank account, to draw in a case of an emergency! Say, for hard times By Body Fluids we mean sweat, saliva, semen, the mucus, lymph, etc. The original source is the food and our drink. Their sudden or prolonged deficiency can lead to the immediate lack of blood eg Sauna or the emesis (deliberate vomiting) yogic techniques. Their accumulation causes swelling.

The Functions of the Internal Organs

This is about another system of the Traditional Chinese Medicine Theory, according to which the functions of internal vital organs control, store and affect the Vital Substances. In Western Medicine internal organs mostly have an anatomical role, while in Chinese Medicine besides their anatomical role, possess some relationships with our feelings, body tissues, sensory organs, mental strength, etc. For example, the Heart governs Blood, is related to Joy and manifested in facial complexion, while the Liver controls the menstrual cycle, is associated with anger and manifests in nails, etc.

The Causes of Disease

Traditional Chinese Medicine sets balance as the key to health. Balance in work out exercise, at rest, in our diet, in our sexual activity, climate and more. When prolonged period overturned the balance occurs disharmony. The disharmony is manifested in weakness. According to Chinese medicine, diseases may have to do with our inner world or with the external pathogenic conditions in which we live or just to other causes.

Internal causes may be our emotions such as fear, joy, sadness, shock, excessive thinking, worry, anger. Each one of these emotions infects the Qi affecting a specific organ, eg Worry affects the Spleen, Grief affects the Lungs, etc.

External causes may be the climatic factors such as cold, heat/ fire, the summer heat, dampness, dryness and wind. The Chinese Medicine here again uses a poetic term and refers to them as "The 6 Demons" because they try to intrude inside the human like Demons.

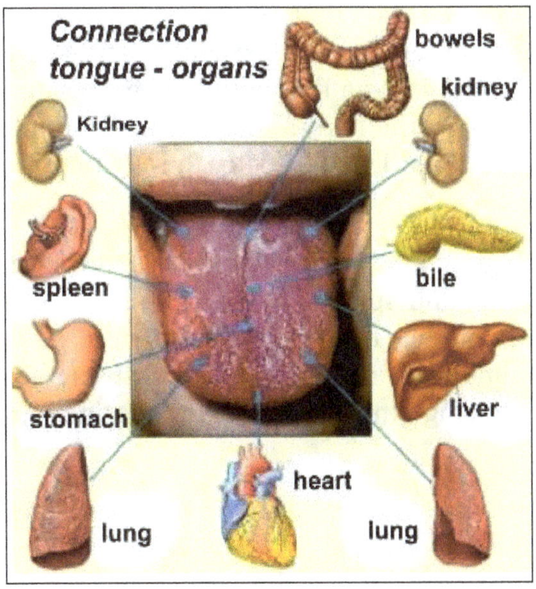

Other causes of disease are a poor constitution/heredity, overexertion in physical/ mental work and exercise, excessive sexual activity, poor dietary hobbits, trauma, parasites & poisoning, incorrect treatment.

Sexual activity for example, according to the book "Classic of the simple girl", must be exercised in accordance with the age of the man or the woman and the average state of health. eg for men 30 years old every day, 40 years old every 3 days, 50 years old every 5 days, etc. Of course this should not be taken for granted, but only as a larger point of view.

According to Chinese Medicine, male ejaculation has a relationship with the loss of Essence which is housed at Kidneys. On the contrary, women have less Essence loss, as it has to do with the Uterus. Of course, women experience a much greater loss of Essence during the period and birth.

Qigong

Qigong means "skill in managing the Breath of Life". It's an ancient healing art utilizing meditation, movement exercises, self-massage, and special healing techniques to regulate internal functions of the human body. Qigong is a Branche of Traditional Chinese Medicine (TCM) along with acupuncture & moxibustion, herbology, and tuina (massage). Its practice can promote, preserve, circulate, balance and store Qi (or"chi", vital energy) within the body to achieve health and longevity.

Archeological finds in China depict Qigong movements at least three thousand years ago, and some believe it goes back 8,000. years. The 3500 year old Internal Medicine Classic refers to "ancient ones" who understood Qi thousands of years earlier. Other old texts suggest Qigong is the "grandfather" of basic theories of Chinese medicine and other healing modalities in Asia that employ the concepts of Qi and its circular pulsation of Yin and Yang in the body's meridians. (Examples: ki is the Japanese word for Qi, Do is the word for Tao: Ai-ki-do, Rei-ki, Jin Shin-do are all derivative schools.)

The major schools of Qigong are Taoist, Buddhist, and Confucian. The three major types are martial, medical, and spiritual, with Taoism being famous for its medical styles. Although there are literally hundreds, if not thousands, of different styles of Qigong, most have the common purpose of relaxing and strengthening the body, improving mental capacity, nurturing innate potential, promoting longevity, and preventing or treating disease.

For these reasons, Qigong is called the "Chinese Miracle Exercise." The better known Tai Chi Chuan is actually a series of short qigong movements strung together to create a longer "form". An estimated 100 million people around the world today practice

Qigong on a daily basis for its many benefits, making it possibly the world's most popular health exercise.

Mechanism of Action According to its Own Theory

What is Qi? It is the Life Force (bio-force, or matrix of primal energy) that underlies all existence, from subatomic particles to galaxies to empty space itself. Within humans it is the very substance of our aliveness that pulsates at varying rates within our vital organs and cells. Different qualities of qi define and regulate different biological functions, just as a stem cell differentiates into specialized functions.

Qi is NOT mechanical energy, it is the intelligent mind substance that crystallizes into our thoughts, feelings, sensations, desires, and cells. It's the motive force of DNA replication and immune system function. Qi is the functional level of the body's innate intelligence.

Qigong shares the same philosophical foundation as Traditional Chinese Medicine (which is actually modern) with its theories of Qi and Blood, Yin/Yang, Meridians & Zang-Fu Organs, Five Elements, and the pathogenesis of disease. It also embodies the older Classical Chinese Medicine which focuses on the alchemical transformations between Shen (mind), Qi (energy), and Jing (body essence) and the shamanic concept of the Five Jing Shen ("vital organ souls") that govern one's health. Beyond the overlap of theory, the methods of Qigong differ from those of acupuncture, herbology, and massage.

When Qi becomes deficient or excessive, stagnant or blocked in different parts of the body, or unable to ward off pathogenic factors, a pattern of imbalance is set up that can lead to disease. Imbalances in Qi can occur as a result of improper diet, over strain, stress, lack of physical exercise, traumatic injury, toxins, environmental factors (wind, cold, summer heat, dampness, dryness), or the seven emotions (anger, worry, sadness, grief, fear, fright, joy). When the body?s natural equilibrium is overcome by any of these factors, disease can occur.

One type of qigong therapy employs "external qi emission".

The qigong healer may tap into either his personal or universal energy which is then focused and radiated into the patient's body lying on a table or while sitting. This alters the energetic matrix of the patient's meridians, and causes their physical body to be regenerated. The patient may feel a gentle warmth or tingling begin to flow in different parts of the body. Depending on the skill of the healer, it can be used with great success on anything from mild headache to broken bones to sexual dysfunction as well as chronic illnesses such as cancer and aids. Some healers can work at a distance, even hundreds of miles away.

The second type is for a patient to self-practice qigong. The patient is taught how to do qigong movements and meditations that will benefit their particular condition. Some are specifically designed for different illnesses, i.e. asthma, a special anti-cancer walk or for joint disease, and others are meant to balance the qi of summer, winter, or the heart or lung meridian, etc. All are easily performed even by the elderly or by people in a weak condition. The patient usually feels improvement immediately and a general sense of well-being.

The powerful Qi meditation methods known as "neigong" create "internal qi movements" using the mind to flow qi in the meridians. Most famous is the "microcosmic orbit", which circulates qi up the spine and down the front of the body. Others might use sub-vocal sound frequencies focused on the vital organs (the "six healing sounds"), or by evoking postive feeling states (the "inner smile"). There is even a sexual qigong for redirecting sexual qi to alleviate impotence, PMS, and stimulate the production of hormonal pre-cursors in the bone marrow.

The self-practice approach requires self-discipline on the part of the patient, but because the patient is taught how to take responsibility for their own healing it generally produces the most effective and lasting results. Once the patient learns to generate "qi" within themselves, the results are not limited to self-healing. You may continue to practice the qigong to achieve ever higher levels of wellness and spiritual awareness. Qigong is so simple yet powerful that many healers use qigong to repair themselves from "healer burnout".

Biologic Mechanism of Action

The physiological effects of Qigong have been extensively scientifically studied in the past twenty years. The Computerized Qigong Database (Qigong Institute) has over 1300 studies. Qigong has been shown to decrease blood pressure, decrease oxygen consumption, increase respiratory efficiency, improve cardiovacular functioning, alter and integrate brain wave patterns, decrease stress hormone levels, and improve cellular and humoral immunity.

These changes are characteristic of effects on central and autonomic nervous systems, hormones, and neurotransmitters. The overall relaxation response is believed to play a significant role in the mitigation of the devastating effects of stress, and the prevention and treatment of illness.

There are seven aspects of emitted qi that have been quantified scientifically. Qi emission resulted in significant changes in infrasound, electromagnetic, static electricity, infrared radiation, gamma rays, particle and wave flows, organic ion flows, and light. Most dramatic were human infrasonic frequencies that leaped from 60 MHz to 400,000. MHz during qi emission.

In experiments on externally emitted qi from Qigong masters on various biological substrates and chemical compounds, emitted Qi was found to affect DNA synthesis and structure, protein synthesis, artificial cell membranes, chemical reactions, and polarized light beams. In similar experiments involving long-distance Qi emission and its effects on molecular structures, evidence was found to suggest the existence of such a phenomenon.

Research into emitted Qi is still in its infancy, but it is rapidly expanding our knowledge of human biomagnetic energy. Study of emitted Qi on biological systems has the potential to unsettle the foundation of modern science and thinking. Qigong does not appear to behave entirely according to the laws of linear physics, but rather to the advanced concepts of quantum and chaos theories.

Forms of Therapy

Internal (self-practice) and external (qi emission) qigong are the two broad divisions.

Internal Qigong consists of meditation and movement exercises which are practiced by individuals to regulate their own Qi. External Qigong is performed by a trained Qigong practitioner to detect and correct imbalances in the circulation of Qi in another person.

Indications and Reasons for Referral

Most older children and adults can learn to practice simple Qigong to increase their sense of well being, decrease stress, improve health, prevent illness, and especially to treat chronic and difficult conditions. Qigong is a valuable adjunct to Western medicine in that it supports a pro-active, preventative approach to health.

Qigong therapy alone is not appropriate for acute or emergency situations unless the Qigong therapist is highly skilled and experienced.

Common reasons for referring someone to Qigong instruction or therapy:

- Management of chronic illness.
- Wellness promotion/preventative medicine.
- Stress management.
- Inability of Western medicine to clearly diagnose an illness or condition i.e. strange or bizarre symptoms that don?t conform to any known Western pattern of disease.
- Patient requests ?holistic or natural? treatment options.
- Unacceptable risk (to patient or physician) of proposed medical intervention.
- Terminal illness: palliative or therapeutic stages.

Research Base

Most of the research on Qigong in the past 30 years are in abstracts in proceedings from international scientific meetings or published in Chinese. Many are now available through the Qigong Institute research database.

Evidence Based

Several studies suggest Qigong can reduce both systolic and diastolic high blood pressure, decrease the amount of medication required to stabilize hypertension. It reduces excessive responses to stress and improves the function of the hypothalamic-pituitary-adrenal axis.

In an impressive twenty-two year controlled study of 244 hypertensive patients, Qigong practice was shown to decrease overall mortality (19.3% Qigong vs. 41.7% controls), decrease the incidence (18 % Qigong vs. 41 % control) and mortality for stroke (13.9 % Qigong vs. 24.7 % controls), improve control of systolic and diastolic blood pressure, and help reduce antihypertensive medication dosages (47.7 % of the Qigong group in contrast with an increased dosage requirement in 30.85 % of the control group). Qigong also helps offset cardiovascular lesions such as progressive retinopathy and abnormal ECG findings.

Studies suggest Qigong affects hormonal balance, decreasing estradiol levels in hypertensive men and increasing estradiol and testosterone levels in post-menopausal women. It improves left ventricular function, increases cardiac output, and decreases peripheral vascular resistance in patients with essential hypertension and coronary heart disease.

Hemodialysis patients reported subjective improvements in appetite, increased frequency of bowel movements, increase in general well-being and physical strength, improved sexual activity, and sleep quality.

Basic Science

The existence and measurement of Qi has been the object of many studies. Seto et al. measured an extraordinarily large magnetic field (10-3 gauss) emanating from the palms of three individuals emitting Qi. This is one thousand times stronger than the known, naturally occurring human bio-magnetic field (10-6 gauss). The frequency of this unusual magnetic wave was 4 to 10 Hz.

Chien et al. documented the effects of emitted Qi on human fibroblast cell growth, DNA synthesis, protein synthesis and boar sperm respiration.

Studies suggest several possible mechanisms for the physiological effects of Qigong. Emitted Qi is able to affect RNA and DNA UV absorption, change artificial phospholipid membranes, and alter molecular compositions of non-living substances similar to those found in the body. Similar results at long distances defy our current understanding of physical laws.

The effects of Qigong on the nervous system have been well studied. The Qigong state is different from the waking state, resting with eyes closed, drowsiness, sleep, or any state in between. EEG studies show slowing of alpha peak frequency and increase in alpha-1 (8-10 Hz) components in the anterior-frontal regions.

Qigong meditation with active abdominal breathing is a method common to many schools. In one study, this was found to improve ventilatory efficiency for O_2 and CO_2 by about 20%.

Risk and Safety

Qigong enjoys an enviable and remarkable safety profile, but is not without possible side effects. Side effects are infrequent and are usually not due to the techniques themselves, but rather to incorrect practice. Patients with acute infections should avoid vigorous types of qigong which may circulate the infected blood. Some White Crane styles with rapid fluttering of limbs have been reported to overstimulate frail individuals, causing nervous breakdown.

Qigong "deviation syndrome" — dizziness, headache, nausea, palpitation, feeling hot or cold, dissociative feeling — is easily corrected by the practitioner with relaxation and correct mind set, body posture, or breathing. Qigong induced psychosis has been described in rare cases with auditory hallucinations and delusions. This is usually self-limited and resolves soon after stopping Qigong. When this fails, an experienced Qigong practitioner or master can help.

Efficacy

The percentage of patients who respond to Qigong vary according to the level of experience and skill of the practitioner. Common estimates of benefits run from 80 to 90 %. With greater length of practice and experience, the benefits appear to increase.

Efficacy is enhanced if people fully commit to practice on a daily basis. In a study of hypertensive patients, the overall mortality rate of people who practiced>3/4 of the timewas 11.2 % compared with 29.3 % in the inconsistent group.

Qigong can infuse Qi into everything that acupuncture needles can, and reach even deeper into the mind-body relationship. This makes it a premier treatment choice for most chronic conditions:

- Hypertension: Benefits include improved blood pressure control (systolic and diastolic), decreased medication use, decreased mortality, decreased incidence and mortality of stroke, offset of the progression of cardiovascular lesions and retinopathy .

- Asthma: Disorders which are affected by emotional components or stress are very amenable to Qigong, which improves respiratory efficiency.
- Allergies: Studies show Qigong can affect the immune system and stabilize the effects of stress and emotions.
- Stress and stress-related disorders: (e.g. fatigue, tension headaches, poor concentration, difficulty.
- Sleeping, problems with appetite, vague aches and pains, etc.) Sitting and moving Qigong are excellent tools to mitigate the devastating effects of stress on the mind, body and spirit.
- Cancer: With experimental data about the effects of Qi on DNA, protein synthesis, chemical reactions, cell growth, the immune system, emotional well-being, and improved quality of life, Qigong should be an integral part of all programs dealing with cancer. Many studies have been presented at scientific meetings about the beneficial effects of Qigong on cancer cells and tumors.
- AIDS: Same reasons as for cancer.
- Gastro-intestinal: Irritable bowel, peptic ulcer disease, poor appetite, constipation, hemorrhoids, etc.
- The effects of Qigong on the functional aspects of digestion are well recognized by research.
- Chronic fatigue/fibromyalgia: These syndromes can be frustrating to treat with Western medicine. Qigong can help these patients rebuild their stores of Qi and balance their energy circulation.
- Diabetes: There is evidence that Qigong can alter hormonal levels in the body. Specific Qigong techniques exist for diabetes mellitus.
- Arthritis: Qigong is often used for arthritis. It appears to benefit rheumatoid as well as osteoarthritis. The exercises are gentle and generally easy to learn.
- Musculoskeletal pains and sports injuries: Acute or chronic musculoskeletal injuries. Best used under the guidance of a trained Qigong practitioner to avoid further injury.
- Low energy states: If Western medical investigations reveal no clear cause for fatigue or low energy states, it is likely due to Qi deficiency.
- Hepatitis: Anecdotal reports of benefits. Some schools have specific Qigong techniques for hepatitis/liver problems.

Unani Medicine

Unani medicine is popular in South Asian countries and its use is growing in other parts of the world. It has now become part of the mainstream system of medicine in Bangladesh, India, Islamic Republic of Iran, Pakistan, and others.

Unani medicine encompasses a wide range of practices. Unani regimental therapy includes venesection, cupping, the promotion of diaphoresis and diuresis, Turkish baths, massage, cauterization, purging, emesis, exercise and leeching. Unani diet therapy deals with certain ailments by treating them with specific diets or by regulating the quantity and quality of food. Unani pharmacotherapy uses naturally occurring medicines, mostly herbal medicines and those of animal and mineral origin. Single medicines or their combination in raw form are preferred over compound formulations. Unani physiotherapy uses specific exercise techniques to help balance the homeostasis of the body.

Unani medicine originated in Greece and is primarily based on the principles propounded by the ancient Greek practitioners Hippocrates and Galen. Over the subsequent centuries, a number of Arab and Persian scholars enriched the system, among them Ibn Sina, who is also known as Avicenna. He was an Arab philosopher and physicist, who wrote Kitab-al-shifa (Book of Healing) and the Canon of Medicine. This system, earlier known as "Galenics", later became known as Unani Tibb.

Unani medicine states that disease is a natural process and that symptoms are the reactions of the body to disease. It employs the humoral theory which presupposes the presence of four akhlaat (humours) in the body – dam (blood), balgham (phlegm), safra (yellow bile) and sauda (black bile). Each humour has its own temperament: blood is hot and moist; phlegm is cold and moist; yellow bile is hot and dry; and black bile is cold and dry. According to Unani, if the four main humours and the four primary temperaments (hot, cold, dry, moist) are all in a state of mutual equilibrium, the person is considered healthy.

In Unani medicine, six key factors are evaluated in relation to health. These six factors are called "al-umoor al-tabiyah". Each has a close relation to, and a direct bearing on, the state of health of an individual. Therefore, it is necessary for a Unani medicine practitioner to take all these factors into consideration in order to arrive at a correct diagnosis and decide how to treat the ailment.

Concepts of the Stages of Digestion

According to the Unani system of medicine, there are four stages of digestion.

- Gastric digestion followed by intestinal digestion, when food is turned into chyme and chyle and carried to the liver.

- Hepatic digestion, when chyle is converted into the four humours in varying quantities, blood being the largest. Thus, the blood that leaves the liver is intermixed with the other three humours; phlegm, yellow bile and black bile.
- Vessel digestion, in which every tissue absorbs nutrition by its attractive power and retains it by its retentive power.
- Tissue digestion is the digestive power that, in conjunction with the power of assimilation, converts the nutritive elements into tissue.

The waste material remaining in the humours at this stage is excreted by the expulsive power. Unani practitioners maintain that when any disturbance occurs in the equilibrium of the humours, it causes disease. Therefore the Unani mode of treatment aims to restore the equilibrium of the humours.

States of the Human Body (Haalaat al-jism)

According to Unani medicine practitioners, the states of the body are grouped under three headings:

- Health, in which all the functions of the body operate normally;
- Disease, the opposite of health, in which one or more forms or functions of the bodily organs are at fault; and
- Neither health nor disease, where there is neither complete health nor actual disease, such as in the case of elderly individuals or those who are convalescing.

Diseases are of two types, namely simple or complex. A simple disease is one that completes its course without complications. A simple disease may manifest itself in three forms:

- Imbalance of the humours (dyscrasia);
- Structural diseases;
- Diseases of disharmony.

Physical Temperament (Mizaj)

The interaction of the elements produces various states, which in turn determine the temperament of an individual. It is of paramount importance to keep that temperament in mind while prescribing a course of treatment. Each individual has a unique temperament, which may potentially be real equitable, equitable or inequitable. The state of real equitable never occurs in reality, rather it is a theoretical situation in which the temperaments of the four elements used are equal. An equitable temperament denotes an appropriate and required amount of compatible temperaments. An inequitable temperament results from an inappropriate distribution of temperaments for the requirements of the individual's condition.

Prevention of Disease

Unani medicine has long recognized the influence of surroundings and ecological conditions on the state of health of human beings. It has a theory on the six essential prerequisites for the prevention of disease and it places great emphasis on the maintenance of a proper ecological balance and on keeping water, food and air free from all pollution. These prerequisites, known as al-asbab al-sitta al-dharuriya (six essentials) may be briefly explained as follows:

- Al-hawaa (air): Good, clean air is necessary for health and many diseases are said to occur owing to changes in the air. Abu Sina, the famous Unani medicine practitioner, said that a change of environment can relieve patients of many diseases. Abu Sina also emphasized the need for open, airy houses with proper ventilation and for playgrounds and gardens in the cities so that everyone could get plenty of fresh air to allow for maintenance of a proper ecological cycle;

- Al-maakool wa al-mashroob (food and drink): Food should be fresh and free from putrefaction and pathogens. Drinking water should also be pure;

- Harakat wa sukoon al-baden (physical exercise and repose): To maintain positive health and fitness, the body requires both exercise and rest. Inflammation and fractures require total rest for an optimum healing. On the other hand, afflictions such as paralysis demand specific types of movement. Several exercises help muscles to grow and ensure increased blood supply and proper functioning of the excretory system. Exercise also keeps the heart and liver in good condition.

- Mental exertion and repose: Psychological factors such as happiness, sorrow, and anger are believed to have considerable bearing on the health of the human being. Unani medicine practitioners maintain that certain diseases and disorders, are caused by emotional strain and maladjustment. Therefore, when dealing with such cases, the practitioner should try to take all these factors into account. There is a branch of Unani medicine known as "psychological treatment" that deals with the abovementioned factors, and many diseases are treated by psychological methods. Sometimes this type of treatment is used alone, while at other times it is used in conjunction with various medicines. Unani medicine practitioners have also recognized the effects of music, pleasant company and beautiful scenery.

- Sleep and wakefulness: Normal sleep and wakefulness are essential for health. Sleep is an ideal form of rest; physical as well as mental. Lack of sleep causes dissipation of energies, mental weakness and digestive disturbances.

- Evacuation and retention: Waste products of the body, if not completely and properly excreted, produce disease; The natural means of excretion are diuresis, diaphoresis, vomiting, defecation, excretion through the uterus in the form of menses, excretion through the eyes, ears and nose and respiration. Proper and normal functioning of the excretory processes must be ensured in order to maintain what, in Unani medicine, is considered perfect health. Any disturbance in the normal excretory balances, whether it is excess, diminution or blockage, may lead to disease.

Faculties/Powers (Quwa)

According to Unani medicine there are three kinds of powers: psychic (natural) power, power of metabolism and power of reproduction.

- Psychic and nervous power is present in the brain and is made up of two other powers: perceptive power, which conveys impressions or sensations, and motive power, which brings about movements as a response to the sensation.

Perceptive power may be external or internal. The external perceptive power recognizes objects outside the body and is served by the five senses. The internal perceptive power operates when perceptions do not come from the outside, but are inferences drawn from external impressions and realizations.

Internal perceptive power uses five other powers:

  - Composite sense, which collects together all external realizations;
  - Imagination, which stores all the materials collected by the composite sense;
  - Conceptualization, which correlates all external realizations and draws conclusions from them;
  - Memory, which stores the conclusions drawn by conceptualization;
  - The modifying faculty, which gives the capacity to explain the same thing in different ways and interprets all internal and external realizations.

- The seat of the power of metabolism is the liver, but the process is active in every tissue of the body. The process of metabolism is conducted by two powers:
  - Nutritive power is developed in the liver from the food eaten and is conveyed to all parts of the body. It is served by four other powers: attractive, retentive, digestive and expulsive;
  - Growing power is responsible for the development and growth of the human organism and is served by three other powers – receptive power, power to retain nutrition and assimilative power.

- Reproduction is accomplished by two powers: generative power and formative power.

Safety Issues

Unani practitioners identify the following safety issues:

- Possible adverse effects of herbal ingredients: Examples of adverse effects of herbal ingredients that have been documented in humans or animals include: allergic, cardiac, hepatic, hormonal, irritant, centralnervous-system and purgative effects, and a range of toxicities.
- The interaction between herbal and conventional medicines: There is limited information available regarding interactions between herbal products and conventional medicines. However, awareness of this issue is increasing and the potential for herbal and conventional medicines interactions should always be considered. Therefore it is important that the patient should give the Unani medicine practitioner full details of all medicines being taken concurrently. Proper precautions and monitoring are required and, if necessary, treatment should be adapted to accommodate for potential herb/conventional drug interaction.

Unani medicine practitioners should practice based on Unani theory and should warn patients when metals, minerals or poisonous substances are included in the prescription or prescribed medicinal formulation. Information regarding the safe use of these substances, signs of potential adverse effects and recommendations for emergency response to these adverse events should be provided. The information collected from the pharmacovigilance system should be learned by Unani practitioners. The dispensers should verify the prescriptions every time, and refer back to the prescribers immediately whenever it is needed.

Native American Healing

Native American (NA) traditional healing is identified by the National Institutes of Health/National Center for Complementary and Alternative Medicine (NCCAM) as a whole medical system that encompasses a range of holistic treatments used by indigenous healers for a multitude of acute and chronic conditions or to promote health and wellbeing.[2] While there are individual tribal differences (i.e., the use of specific healing practices), there are also shared health beliefs and interventional strategies, including a health promotion foundation that embraces bio-psycho-socio-spiritual approaches and traditions. Native Americans in Arizona run each day to greet the dawn, a practice that not only conditions their bodies but also nourishes their spiritual wellbeing. Stories and legends are used to teach positive behaviors as well as the consequences of failing to observe the laws of nature. Herbs, manipulative therapies, ceremonies, and prayer are used in various combinations to prevent and treat illness.

For thousands of years, traditional indigenous medicine have been used to promote health and wellbeing for millions of Native people who once inhabited this continent. Native diets, ceremonies that greet the seasons and the harvests, and the use of native plants for healing purposes have been used to live to promote health by living in harmony with the earth. Increasingly, younger generations of Native people are abandoning these traditions -opportunities for a close connection to the earth – with a resultant increase in disease and impaired health states. Less than 100 years ago, diabetes was almost unheard of among NA. Today diabetes runs rampant through many tribes as they integrate into the mainstream culture and adopt the typical American lifestyle. The consequences of abandonment of traditional practices can be readily seen when comparing the health of younger generations of NA to their living elders who are engaged in traditional health practices.

Symbolic Healing

Ceremonies play an important role in the overall wellbeing of traditional Native American people but the healing potential of this practice is typically unappreciated by allopathic health providers. NA ceremonies involve the patient, the family, and the community in the healing process. Ceremonial gatherings may last for days or weeks; the more people that are present, the greater the healing energy. Through their participation in songs, prayer, music, and dance, the family and community contribute healing energy to the patient.

People of all cultures utilize symbolism found in their various religions and spiritual practices to cope with health problems. NA healing ceremonies rely heavily on a combination of traditional and Christian religious symbols, icons, and ritualistic objects. These symbols cue bio-psycho-social-spiritual healing responses by restoring the harmony necessary for health. Symbolism, whether associated with ceremonies or church services, can be incorporated into their treatment plan to create a powerful healing synergy.

Integrating Indigenous Healing

Today Native Americans frequently combine traditional healing practices with allopathic medicine to promote health and wellbeing. Ceremony, native herbal remedies, and allopathic medications are used side by side. Spiritual treatments are thus an integral part of health promotion and healing in Native American culture.

Yet, the role of spirituality in health promotion and wellness is uncomfortable for many allopathic providers. Advanced practice nurses with their tradition of holism that embraces the bio-psycho-social-spiritual nature of health have an opportunity to suggest new ways to care modeled on traditional NA practices. The inclusion of family and community in treatment plans, decreases the isolation often found in allopathic care. And, thinking about the lack of person-environment harmony and balance may important clues for the diagnostic process.

Curanderismo

Curanderismo is a holistic system of Latin American folk medicine. This type of folk medicine has characteristics specific to the area where it is practiced (Guatemala, Nicaragua, Honduras, Argentina, Mexico, the southwestern region of the United States, etc.). Curanderismo blends religious beliefs, faith, and prayer with the use of herbs, massage, and other traditional methods of healing. Curanderismo can be defined as a set of traditional beliefs, rituals, and practices that address the physical, spiritual, psychological, and social needs of the people who use it.

The Spanish verb curar means to heal. Therefore, curanderismo is translated as a system of healing. The goal of curanderismo is to create a balance between the patient and his or her environment, thereby sustaining health.

The healer who practices curanderismo is referred to as a curandero (male healer) or curandera (female healer). Healing terms vary with the language and culture of the area in which the system is practiced. For example, a female healer in Argentina is called a remedieras.

Curanderismo in Mexico is based on Aztec, Mayan, and Spanish influences. The ancient native cultures believed that a delicate balance existed between health, nature, and religion. Illness occurred when one of these areas was out of balance.

The use of nature's resources was very important to the native cultures. In the fifteenth century, the Huaxtepec garden was developed by the Aztec leader Montezuma I. This garden was a collection of several thousand medicinal plants. The Aztec priests used this garden to perform research on the medicinal properties of the plants.

When the Spanish conquistadors came to Mexico in the sixteenth century, they destroyed the garden and all of the priests' research because the Catholic Church considered these "sciences" to be blasphemous. Although the written knowledge was destroyed, the plant wisdom was remembered, passed down by the native peoples, and became an integral part of curanderismo.

The Spanish missionaries who were sent to the New World introduced the native peoples to the Catholic religion and European healing philosophies. Prayers to Catholic saints were soon integrated into healing rituals. Another doctrine that was passed on to the native peoples by the Europeans was their belief in witchcraft, sorcery, and other superstitions, and the philosophy that illness is often caused by supernatural forces.

As the native and Spanish cultures intermingled over the centuries, a new culture was formed, as was the folk medicine of curanderismo.

Benefits

Curanderismo is used to treat ailments arising from physical, psychological, spiritual, or social conditions. Illness is said to be caused by either natural or supernatural forces.

Naturally caused illness is treated with herbal medicine, massage, and prayer. Much of this illness is thought to be brought about by intense emotions caused by trauma or a specific event. Susto, for example, is an illness that is caused by fright. A startling event such as a fire, earthquake, dog attack, car accident, or death may cause the patient to become ill. Symptoms of susto are insomnia, diarrhea, extreme nervousness, sadness, depression, loss of appetite, loss of brilliance in the eyes, and lack of dreams. The events are thought to dislodge a person's spirit from the body.

Bilis is an ailment that is the result of excessive emotional stress . Bilis is caused by prolonged anger and fear. The ailment is thought to occur when excessive bile is trapped in the system and causes tension, irritability, and loss of appetite.

Empacho and colic are ailments treated by massage and herbs. Empacho is a blocked intestine disease where the intestines are plugged by something indigestible such as chewing gum or unbaked dough. To treat this condition, the curandera performs a massage in which she pulls on the skin of the back just above the coccyx (tailbone). When the skin makes a snapping noise the food has been loosened. Herbal tea is also given to complement the massage.

Colic is caused by excessive coldness of the stomach, and mint is used for such digestive problems.

Supernaturally caused illnesses or conditions are initiated by witchcraft, sorcery, or hexes. Physical symptoms might manifest as nervous breakdowns, paranoia, schizophrenia, depression, or excessive worrying. Supernatural forces can also create social problems. A person who has a streak of bad luck, or who suffers from marital problems, the loss of a job, or car troubles will deem the problem to be caused by a supernatural force. To heal these ailments and remove the hex or problem, the curandera uses rituals, spiritual cleansings, herbs, and prayer.

Prayer is the foundation of curanderismo. Curanderas have strong religious faith and believe that they were given the ability to heal as a gift from God. Curanderas pray to spirits and/or Catholic saints for help in healing their patients, often praying to specific saints for particular conditions.

A traditional healing session may include one or more of the following: spiritual cleansing (limpia), ritual, massage, and/or herbal therapy. Curanderas use a variety of objects in their healing sessions, including herbs and spices, eggs, lemons, flowers, fruits, holy water, pictures of saints, crucifixes, candles, incense, and oils. Each object has a specific purpose.

Holy water is used for protection from negativity or evil spirits. Eggs and lemons are patted on the patient's body to absorb negative energies. Rosemary, basil, and rue branches are brushed on the body to remove negativity.

Candles are burned to absorb negative energy and create a healing environment. Different colored candles are burned for different reasons: red for strength, blue for harmony, pink for good will. Incense is used to purify the room, while garlic and oils are used as protection from negativity and bad spirits.

Iridology

Iridology, also known as iridodiagnosis, is an alternative medicine technique that uses the colors, patterns, and various other properties of the iris to assess an individual's general health. The technique of iridology is based on the belief that each organ in the human body has a corresponding region in the iris. Thus, the premise is that organ functioning can be examined by simply inspecting the iris.

Iridologists generally utilize cameras, flashlights, and microscopes to examine the patient's iris in order to detect tissue change, stromal irregularities and pigment patterns. The results are then compared with an iris chart, which helps in correlating the various parts of the human body with different zones in the iris.

A typical iris chart usually divides the iris into approximately 90 zones, each corresponding to a different part of the human body. Iridologists believe that the details reflected by the iris are generally the changes in the tissues of the corresponding body organelle.

According to proponents of this therapy, iridology is not meant to diagnose illness, but rather to detect impaired organ functions attributable to environmental toxins, poor nutrition, and fatigue.

For iridologists, color variations in the iris (sparkles and rings) carry specific significance and can even indicate whether a suspected condition is acute/inflammatory, chronic/inflammatory, or allergic.

Some iridologists further divide organ system dysfunction by iris color. They believe that lymphatic-related disease is associated with a blue or blue-gray iris and that these individuals are prone to atopic conditions; hematogenous-related pathology is linked to brown-eyed individuals who are more prone to anemia and endocrine disorders; biliary disease is associated with both blue and brown irises, and is indicative of gastric deficiencies.

Iridology was used as early as the 17th century in Europe, but the practice gained notice in the United States only in the latter half of the 20th century. Despite its long history, there are scarce scientific data to support iridology's utility.

Science

Out of the four of conditions most commonly assessed by practitioners of iridology (hypertension, cancer, gallbladder disease, and kidney disease), only hypertension earned a strength-of-evidence grade of "C," while the remaining three conditions ended with very weak showings of "D" levels.

In one study, researchers explored the overlapping of tumor necrosis factor-alpha (TNF-alpha), hypertension, and specific variations of iris constitution. Eighty-seven Korean patients with known hypertension were compared with 79 Korean participants with no known BP concerns.

Individuals were evaluated on iris characteristics, BP, and the presence or absence of the TNF-alpha genotype. The study results did not show a statistically significant difference in the genotype and the presence of hypertension, but there was a definite elevation in the hypertensive patients with the iris characteristic denoting cardio-renal connective-tissue weakness.

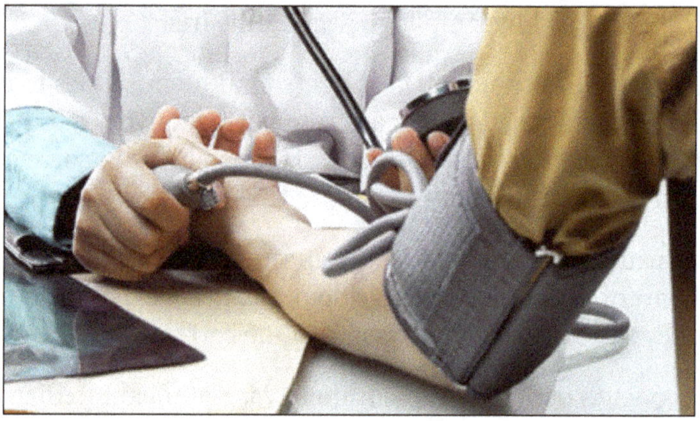

In another study of the same patient population, researchers examined study participants for a correlation of iris characteristics and the presence or absence of apolipoprotein-E (apoE). There is a well-established relationship between this genotype and vascular diseases, including hypertension. In a blind study, patients were examined by iris pattern and then testing for the apoE genotype. There was a significant correlation between iris type and hypertension, and an increased percentage of apoE presence in those same hypertensive patients.

Both these studies were not large enough to support the practice of iridology. Further trials with larger study populations are needed.

Studies on the practice have also typically focused on the potential utility of iridology as a screening tool for cancer. One trial examined age- and gender-matched participants for the possibility of colorectal cancer. Twenty-nine patients with known diagnoses of this disease were matched with 29 healthy patients.

The researchers presented photographic slides of each participant's eyes to two trained iridology practitioners. At the end of the study, the presence of cancer was detected in only 50%-53% of patients, proving no better than random chance.

In another trial exploring iridology and cancer detection, 68 patients with known cancer and 42 healthy patients were examined by a single, experienced iridologist. With no other information than the visualization of the iris, the practitioner correctly detected only three cases of cancer.

Safety and Interactions

Because of the noninterventional nature of this practice, there are no contraindications for use. In the United States, there are many organizations for training and education in iridology, but the practice is not regulated by the health-care industry.

Reiki

Reiki is hands-on natural healing using the universal life force energy. The term comes from the Japanese words "rei," meaning universal, and "ki," which means vital life force energy that flows through all living things. Reiki, an abundant, gentle spiritual energy is not tied to any specific religion or nationality.

Reiki, which is used all over the world in places including hospitals and hospices, was developed by a Japanese man named Mikao Usui in the early 1900s. It aids in healing by helping people become energetically balanced physically, emotionally, mentally and spiritually.

The Reiki practitioner is the conduit between the patient and the source of the universal life force energy; the energy flows through the practitioner's energy field and through her hands to the patient. (The energy does not come from the practitioner; rather it comes through the practitioner from the universal source. There is no energy drain on the practitioner).

Reiki treatments typically last about 50 minutes. During the treatment the patient lies on a massage table, fully clothed. The Reiki practitioner gently places her hands palms down on or just above the patient's body in specific energy locations and uses a series of 12 to 15 different hand positions. The length of time that the practitioner leaves her hands in each position is determined by the flow of energy through her hands at each location. There is no pressure, massage or manipulation.

The patient experiences the energy as sensations such as heat, tingling or pulsing where the practitioner has placed her hands. Sometimes, the sensations are felt moving through the body; some people do not perceive any change at all. Most people feel very relaxed and peaceful, and many fall asleep during the treatment.

Benefits of Receiving Reiki

According to the National Center for Complementary and Alternative Medicine, people use Reiki for relaxation, stress reduction and symptom relief, in efforts to improve overall health and well-being. A Reiki treatment may do the following:

- Bring about a peaceful, deep state of relaxation.
- Dissolve energy blockages and tension.
- Detoxify the body.
- Support the well-being of a person receiving traditional medical treatments that are debilitating (e.g., chemotherapy, radiation, surgery, kidney dialysis).
- Supply universal life force energy to the body.
- Stimulate the body's immune system.
- Help to relieve pain.
- Stimulate tissue and bone healing after injury or surgery.
- Increase the vibrational frequency on physical, mental, emotional and spiritual levels.

Reiki is Used for the Treatment

Reiki is not specific to any particular type of disease or condition. Because it works on the entire self – mind, body and emotions – and because it is universal life force energy, it may be successful in all types of physical, emotional, mental and spiritual healing. Pets and other animals respond positively to Reiki healing as well.

Reiki practitioners in our Center for Integrative Medicine help patients to prepare for surgery, which may help boost recovery afterward. Our Reiki practitioners see patients for the following conditions, among others:

- Cancer,
- Chronic pain,
- Infertility,
- Digestive problems,
- Parkinson's disease,
- Stress-related diseases,
- Psychological illnesses.

References

- Aromatherapy-the-doctor-of-natural-harmony-of-body—mind, drug-development: ijddr.in, Retrieved 30 June, 2019
- Applied-kinesiology, medicine, divisions-diagnostics-and-procedures: encyclopedia.com, Retrieved 10 April, 2019
- Magnetic-field-therapy-overview, pain-management: webmd.com, Retrieved 24 April, 2019
- Revisiting-reflexology-Concept-evidence-current-practice-and-practitioner-training-282575032: researchgate.net, Retrieved 20 July, 2019
- Qigong-therapy-as-alternativecomplementary-medicine: healingtaousa.com, Retrieved 26 August, 2019
- Curanderismo, encyclopedias-almanacs-transcripts-and-maps: encyclopedia.com, Retrieved 31 August, 2019
- Iridology-detecting-impaired-organ-function-with-the-iris, alternative-meds-update: clinicaladvisor.com, Retrieved 11 June, 2019

5

Herbal Remedies

Herbal medicines are made from plants which are believed to have therapeutic properties. Some of such herbs include aloe vera, ginger, licorice, panax ginseng, etc. This chapter discusses in detail the theories and methodologies related to herbal medicine.

An herb is a plant or plant part used for its scent, flavor, or therapeutic properties. Herbal medicines are one type of dietary supplement. They are sold as tablets, capsules, powders, teas, extracts, and fresh or dried plants. People use herbal medicines to try to maintain or improve their health.

Many people believe that products labeled "natural" are always safe and good for them. This is not necessarily true. Herbal medicines do not have to go through the testing that drugs do. Some herbs, such as comfrey and ephedra, can cause serious harm. Some herbs can interact with prescription or over-the-counter medicines.

Aloe Vera

The Aloe vera plant has been known and used for centuries for its health, beauty, medicinal and skin care properties. The name Aloe vera derives from the Arabic word "Alloeh" meaning "shining bitter substance," while "vera" in Latin means "true." 2000 years ago, the Greek scientists regarded Aloe vera as the universal panacea. The Egyptians called Aloe "the plant of immortality." Today, the Aloe vera plant has been used for various purposes in dermatology.

Aloe vera has been used for medicinal purposes in several cultures for millennia: Greece, Egypt, India, Mexico, Japan and China. Egyptian queens Nefertiti and Cleopatra used it as part of their regular beauty regimes. Alexander the Great, and Christopher Columbus used it to treat soldiers' wounds.

The first reference to Aloe vera in English was a translation by John Goodyew in A.D. 1655 of Dioscorides' Medical treatise De Materia Medica. By the early 1800s, Aloe vera was in use as a laxative in the United States, but in the mid-1930s, a turning point occurred when it was successfully used to treat chronic and severe radiation dermatitis.

Plant

The botanical name of Aloe vera is Aloe barbadensis miller. It belongs to Asphodelaceae (Liliaceae) family, and is a shrubby or arborescent, perennial, xerophytic, succulent, pea- green color plant. It grows mainly in the dry regions of Africa, Asia, Europe and America.

Anatomy

The plant has triangular, fleshy leaves with serrated edges, yellow tubular flowers and fruits that contain numerous seeds. Each leaf is composed of three layers: 1) An inner clear gel that contains 99% water and rest is made of glucomannans, amino acids, lipids, sterols and vitamins. 2) The middle layer of latex which is the bitter yellow sap and contains anthraquinones and glycosides. 3) The outer thick layer of 15–20 cells called as rind which has protective function and synthesizes carbohydrates and proteins. Inside the rind are vascular bundles responsible for transportation of substances such as water (xylem) and starch (phloem).

- Active components with its properties: Aloe vera contains 75 potentially active constituents: vitamins, enzymes, minerals, sugars, lignin, saponins, salicylic acids and amino acids.
- Vitamins: It contains vitamins A (beta-carotene), C and E, which are antioxidants. It also contains vitamin B12, folic acid, and choline. Antioxidant neutralizes free radicals.
- Enzymes: It contains 8 enzymes: aliiase, alkaline phosphatase, amylase, bradykinase, carboxypeptidase, catalase, cellulase, lipase, and peroxidase. Bradykinase helps to reduce excessive inflammation when applied to the skin topically, while others help in the breakdown of sugars and fats.
- Minerals: It provides calcium, chromium, copper, selenium, magnesium, manganese, potassium, sodium and zinc. They are essential for the proper functioning of various enzyme systems in different metabolic pathways and few are antioxidants.
- Sugars: It provides monosaccharides (glucose and fructose) and polysaccharides: (glucomannans/polymannose). These are derived from the mucilage layer of the plant and are known as mucopolysaccharides. The most prominent monosaccharide is mannose-6-phosphate, and the most common polysaccharides are called glucomannans [beta-(1,4)-acetylated mannan]. Acemannan, a prominent glucomannan has also been found. Recently, a glycoprotein with antiallergic properties, called alprogen and novel anti-inflammatory compound, C-glucosyl chromone, has been isolated from Aloe vera gel.

- Anthraquinones: It provides 12 anthraquinones, which are phenolic compounds traditionally known as laxatives. Aloin and emodin act as analgesics, antibacterials and antivirals.
- Fatty acids: It provides 4 plant steroids; cholesterol, campesterol, β-sisosterol and lupeol. All these have anti-inflammatory action and lupeol also possesses antiseptic and analgesic properties.
- Hormones: Auxins and gibberellins that help in wound healing and have anti-inflammatory action.
- It provides 20 of the 22 human required amino acids and 7 of the 8 essential amino acids. It also contains salicylic acid that possesses anti-inflammatory and antibacterial properties. Lignin, an inert substance, when included in topical preparations, enhances penetrative effect of the other ingredients into the skin. Saponins that are the soapy substances form about 3% of the gel and have cleansing and antiseptic properties.

Mechanism of Actions

- Healing properties: Glucomannan, a mannose-rich polysaccharide, and gibberellin, a growth hormone, interacts with growth factor receptors on the fibroblast, thereby stimulating its activity and proliferation, which in turn significantly increases collagen synthesis after topical and oral Aloe vera. Aloe gel not only increased collagen content of the wound but also changed collagen composition (more type III) and increased the degree of collagen cross linking. Due to this, it accelerated wound contraction and increased the breaking strength of resulting scar tissue. An increased synthesis of hyaluronic acid and dermatan sulfate in the granulation tissue of a healing wound following oral or topical treatment has been reported.
- Effects on skin exposure to UV and gamma radiation: Aloe vera gel has been reported to have a protective effect against radiation damage to the skin. Exact role is not known, but following the administration of aloe vera gel, an antioxidant protein, metallothionein, is generated in the skin, which scavenges hydroxyl radicals and prevents suppression of superoxide dismutase and glutathione peroxidase in the skin. It reduces the production and release of skin keratinocyte-derived immunosuppressive cytokines such as interleukin-10 (IL-10) and hence prevents UV-induced suppression of delayed type hypersensitivity.
- Anti-inflammatory action: Aloe vera inhibits the cyclooxygenase pathway and reduces prostaglandin E2 production from arachidonic acid. Recently, the novel anti-inflammatory compound called C-glucosyl chromone was isolated from gel extracts.

- Effects on the immune system: Alprogen inhibit calcium influx into mast cells, thereby inhibiting the antigen-antibody-mediated release of histamine and leukotriene from mast cells. In a study on mice that had previously been implanted with murine sarcoma cells, acemannan stimulates the synthesis and release of interleukin-1 (IL-1) and tumor necrosis factor from macrophages in mice, which in turn initiated an immune attack that resulted in necrosis and regression of the cancerous cells. Several low-molecular-weight compounds are also capable of inhibiting the release of reactive oxygen free radicals from activated human neutrophils.

- Laxative effects: Anthraquinones present in latex are a potent laxative. It increases intestinal water content, stimulates mucus secretion and increases intestinal peristalsis.

- Antiviral and antitumor activity: These actions may be due to indirect or direct effects. Indirect effect is due to stimulation of the immune system and direct effect is due to anthraquinones. The anthraquinone aloin inactivates various enveloped viruses such as herpes simplex, varicella zoster and influenza. In recent studies, a polysaccharide fraction has shown to inhibit the binding of benzopyrene to primary rat hepatocytes, thereby preventing the formation of potentially cancer-initiating benzopyrene-DNA adducts. An induction of glutathione S-transferase and an inhibition of the tumor-promoting effects of phorbol myristic acetate has also been reported which suggest a possible benefit of using aloe gel in cancer chemoprevention.

- Moisturizing and anti-aging effect: Mucopolysaccharides help in binding moisture into the skin. Aloe stimulates fibroblast which produces the collagen and elastin fibers making the skin more elastic and less wrinkled. It also has cohesive effects on the superficial flaking epidermal cells by sticking them together, which softens the skin. The amino acids also soften hardened skin cells and zinc acts as an astringent to tighten pores. Its moisturizing effects has also been studied in treatment of dry skin associated with occupational exposure where aloe vera gel gloves improved the skin integrity, decreases appearance of fine wrinkle and decreases erythema. It also has anti-acne effect.

- Antiseptic effect: Aloe vera contains 6 antiseptic agents: Lupeol, salicylic acid, urea nitrogen, cinnamonic acid, phenols and sulfur. They all have inhibitory action on fungi, bacteria and viruses.

Clinical uses: The clinical use of aloe vera is supported mostly by anecdotal data. Though most of these uses are interesting, controlled trials are essential to determine its effectiveness in all the following diseases.

- Uses based on scientific evidence: These uses have been tested in humans or animals. Safety and effectiveness have not always been proven.

- Conditions: Seborrheic dermatitis, psoriasis vulgaris, genital herpes, skin burns, diabetes (type 2), HIV infection, cancer prevention, ulcerative colitis wound healing (results of aloe on wound healing are mixed with some studies reporting positive results and others showing no benefit or potential worsening), pressure ulcers, mucositis, radiation dermatitis, acne vulgaris, lichen planus, frostbite, aphthous stomatitis, and constipation.

- Uses based on tradition or theory: The below uses are based on tradition or scientific theories. They often have not been thoroughly tested in humans, and safety and effectiveness have not always been proven.

  Conditions: Alopecia, bacterial and fungal skin infections, chronic leg wounds, parasitic infections, systemic lupus erythematosus, arthritis and tic douloureux.

Side Effects

- Topical: It may cause redness, burning, stinging sensation and rarely generalized dermatitis in sensitive individuals. Allergic reactions are mostly due to anthraquinones, such as aloin and barbaloin. It is best to apply it to a small area first to test for possible allergic reaction.

- Oral: Abdominal cramps, diarrhea, red urine, hepatitis, dependency or worsening of constipation. Prolonged use has been reported to increase the risk of colorectal cancer. Laxative effect may cause electrolyte imbalances (low potassium levels).

- Contraindication: Contraindicated in cases of known allergy to plants in the Liliaceae family.

- Pregnancy and breastfeeding: Oral aloe is not recommended during pregnancy due to theoretical stimulation of uterine contractions, and in breastfeeding mothers, it may sometime causes gastrointestinal distress in the nursing infant.

- Interactions: Application of aloe to skin may increase the absorption of steroid creams such as hydrocortisone. It reduces the effectiveness and may increases the adverse effects of digoxin and digitoxin, due to its potassium lowering effect. Combined use of Aloe vera and furosemide may increase the risk of potassium depletion. It decreases the blood sugar levels and thus may interact with oral hypoglycemic drugs and insulin.

Thus, though Aloe vera has wide spectrum of the properties and uses, some of them could be myths and some of them could be real magic. In future, controlled studies are required to prove the effectiveness of Aloe vera under various conditions.

Bach Flower Remedies

Bach Flower Remedies are thought to help balance emotional state and are commonly recommended by practitioners for psychological problems and pain. We assessed whether Bach Flower Remedies (BFRs) are safe and efficacious for these indications by performing.

Methods

You searched MEDLINE, Embase, AMED, and the Cochrane Library from inception until June 2008 and performed a hand-search of references from relevant key articles. For efficacy, we included all prospective studies with a control group. For safety, we also included retrospective, observational studies with more than 30 subjects. Two authors abstracted data and determined risk of bias using a recognised rating system of trial quality.

Results

Four randomised controlled trials (RCTs) and two additional retrospective, observational studies were identified and included in the review. Three RCTs of BFRs for students with examination anxiety, and one RCT of BFRs for children with attention-deficit hyperactivity disorder (ADHD) showed no overall benefit in comparison to placebo. Due to the number and quality of the studies the strength of the evidence is low or very low. We did not find any controlled prospective studies regarding the efficacy of BFRs for pain. Only four of the six studies included for safety explicitly reported adverse events.

Most of the available evidence regarding the efficacy and safety of BFRs has a high risk of bias. We conclude that, based on the reported adverse events in these six trials, BFRs are probably safe. Few controlled prospective trials of BFRs for psychological problems and pain exist. Our analysis of the four controlled trials of BFRs for examination anxiety and ADHD indicates that there is no evidence of benefit compared with a placebo intervention.

Bach flower remedies (BFRs) are a widely-available, popular form of complementary and alternative medicine (CAM) developed in the 1930s by the British physician Dr Edward Bach. Bach devoted his life to the discovery of 38 remedies that correspond to 38 negative emotional states. Bach believed in a truly holistic form of emotional healing; BFRs are believed to assist the body in healing itself by providing "a positive emotional state that is conducive to the restoration of a healthy equilibrium and by acting to catalyze an individual's own internal resources for maintaining balance". According to Bach, the restoration of balance could be used for treating any medical condition, however BFRs are commonly used for psychological problems and stress.

Table: The Bach flower remedies and their indications.

Agrimony	Mental torture behind a cheerful face.
Aspen	Fear of unknown things.
Beech	Intolerance, perfectionist.
Centazry	The inability to say 'no'.
Cerato	Lack of trust in one's own decisions.
Cherry Plum	Fear of the mind giving way, fear of losing control.
Chestnut Bud	Failure to learn from mistakes.
Chicory	Selfish, possessive love, needs the appreciation of others.
Clematis	Dreaming of the future without working in the present, absentminded.
Crab Apple	The cleansing remedy, also for self-hatred, poor body image.
Elm	Overwhelmed by responsibility, pressures of work.
Gentian	Discouragement after a setback, pessimism.
Gorse	Hopelessness and despair.
Heather	Self-centredness and self-concern.
Holly	Hatred, envy and jealousy, feels victimized.
Honeysuckle	Living in the past, overwhelming nostalgia for the past.
Hornbeam	Procrastination, tiredness at the thought of doing something.
Impatiens	Impatience.
Larch	Lack of confidence, competent but fear failure.
Mimulus	Fear of known things, shy, nervous personality.
Mustard	Deep gloom for no reason.
Oak	The plodder who keeps going past the point of exhaustion.
Olive	Exhaustion following mental or physical effort.
Pine	Guilt, self-blame.
Red Chestnut	Over-concern for the welfare of loved ones.
Rock Rose	Terror and fright, useful for nightmares.
Rock Water	Self-denial, rigidity and self-repression.
Scleranthus	Inability to choose between alternatives.
Star of Bethlehem	Shock, loss, bereavement, trauma.
Sweet Chestnut	Extreme mental anguish, when everything has been tried and there is no light left.
Vervain	Over-enthusiasm, perfectionism.
Vine	Dominance and inflexibility.
Walnut	Protection from change and unwanted influences, birth, puberty, divorce.
Water Violet	Pride and aloofness.
White Chestnut	Unwanted thoughts and mental arguments, unwanted thoughts, unable to concentrate.
Wild Oat	Uncertainty over one's direction in life.

Wild Rose	Drifting, resignation, apathy.
Willow	Self-pity and resentment.
Rescue Remedy	Composite remedy consisting of Star of Bethlehem Rock Rose, Cherry Plum and Clementis; for emergencies to combat fear, panic, shock and fear of losing control.

Only flowers that grow naturally in the wild are suitable for preparation. BFRs are prepared in two ways following Bach's precise directions: the sun method and the boiling method. In the sun method, fully opened flower heads still fresh with dew are floated on the surface of pure spring water in a glass bowl and left for a few hours in the sunshine, whereas in the boiling method, used for trees and bushes, the branches and leaves are boiled in water for half an hour. In both methods, the plant matter is removed, and, according to Bach, the water retains the vibrations or energy of the flower. The liquid, called the mother tincture, is filtered and mixed with brandy, which acts as a preservative. The remedies can be taken orally diluted in a glass of water, or applied directly to pulse points such as the wrists, temples and behind the ears. They can be used individually or in combination with up to seven other tinctures. BFRs do not contain pharmacologically relevant remnants of the original flowers and are considered safe to use in combination with other medications, as well as by pregnant women, children, babies and the elderly. However, it has been suggested that BFRs could be dangerous for recovering alcoholics due to their alcohol content.

Bach's 38 flower remedies each address one of the seven psychological causes of illness: fear, uncertainty, insufficient interest in present circumstances, loneliness, oversensitivity to influences and ideas, despondency or despair and overcare for the welfare of others. The individual patient is prescribed particular remedies depending on the acute problem at hand, which should be individually tailored and adjusted during the course of therapy, typically over weeks to months. For example, the flower 'impatiens' is used for impatience and irritability, 'mimulus' for fear of known things, shyness, and timidity, and 'olive' for those that are drained of energy. In addition, some BFRs are categorized as "type" remedies and are specific to a certain character trait or disposition. A person who suffers from overwhelming guilt might be offered pine as a type remedy, and chronically indecisive people could benefit from Scleranthus. Three BFRs are helpful to unblock the energy flow in patients without obvious symptoms: Wild Oat, Holly, and Star of Bethlehem. Because the relief of anxiety is a major factor in pain relief, proponents of BFRs have suggested that BFRs also have the potential to function as a therapeutic agent for pain. "Rescue Remedy", also known as "Five Flower Remedy", is the only combination of BFRs determined by Bach himself and functions as an all purpose emergency agent in situations of acute anxiety or distress. It contains a mixture of star of Bethlehem (Ornithogalum umbellatum), rock rose (Helianthemum nummularium), impatiens (Impatiens glandulifera), cherry plum (Prunus cerasifera), and clematis (Clematis vitalba). Rescue remedy is recommended as a first aid preparation for situations where acute stress is likely to occur.

According to Bach, the remedies work through the life force energy or vibration that is transmitted from the flowers to the tincture. This vibration interacts on a subtle energy level with the individual to rebalance the conscious and unconscious and dissolve old patterns of behavior. By alleviating negative feelings and relieving the underlying emotional and psychological problems of the patient, a physical healing is enabled. Patients sometimes experience a worsening of their symptoms before an improvement, which can manifest as aggravation.

Honey Bee Products

Ever since man has been keeping honeybees, the use of hive products in medicine has been important. Honeybee products, such as honey, bee pollen, propolis, Royal jelly, beeswax, and bee venom, have long been used in traditional medicine. The exact origins of apitherapy can be traced back to ancient Egypt, Greece, and China. Healing properties of honey and other bee products are found in many religious texts including the Veda, Bible, and Quran. In the Old Testament, the land of Israel was often referred to as the "land flowing of milk and honey." The Romans used honey to heal their wounds after battles.

Ethnomedicine, a study of the traditional medicine practiced by various ethnic groups, is a complex multidisciplinary system. It applies the methods of ethnobotany and medical anthropology and constitutes the use of plants and the natural environment. Since ancient times animal products have constituted part of the inventory of medicinal substances used in various cultures. Despite technological developments, bee products along with herbal drugs still occupy a preferential place in a majority of the population in the Third World and terminal patients in the west. Many valuable drugs of today came into use through the study of indigenous remedies. Although ethnomedicine has been the source of healing for people for millennia, it is in the last decade that research interests in ethnomedicine and ethnopharmacy have increased tremendously.

Bee products in their raw form along with crude extracts and purified compounds from them have been shown to exhibit antimicrobial, anti-inflammatory, antioxidative, radio-protective, and tissue-regenerating activities. Some recent studies have revealed that natural honeybee products exhibit immune-modulating properties, inhibit tumor cell growth and metastasis, and induce apoptosis of cancer cells. These bioactive natural products may help manage, among others, cancer, autoimmune diseases, Alzheimer's, Lyme disease, and antibiotic-resistant infections. With the increasing threat of antibiotic-resistant infections and drug over-use, the return to honey bee products as a natural, multipurpose healing therapy makes all the sense in the world.

Panax Ginseng

Panax ginseng is a plant that grows in Korea, northeastern China, and far eastern Siberia. People use the root to make medicine. Do not confuse Panax ginseng with American ginseng, Siberian ginseng, or Panax pseudoginseng.

Panax ginseng is taken by mouth to improve thinking, concentration, memory, Alzheimer's disease, work efficiency, physical stamina, preventing muscle damage from exercise, and athletic endurance.

Some people use Panax ginseng to help them cope with stress and as a general tonic for improving well-being. They sometimes call Panax ginseng an "adaptogen" when it's used in this way.

Panax ginseng is also used for depression, anxiety, general fatigue and chronic fatigue syndrome (CFS), multiple sclerosis, for boosting the immune system, and for fighting particular infections in a lung disease called cystic fibrosis. These infections are caused by a bacterium named Pseudomonas.

Some people use Panax ginseng to treat breast cancer and prevent ovarian cancer, liver cancer, lung cancer, and skin cancer.

Other uses include treatment of anemia, chronic bronchitis, swine flu, prediabetes and diabetes, inflammation of the stomach lining (gastritis), fever, hangover, chronic obstructive pulmonary disease (COPD), HIV/AIDS, fertility problems and sexual dysfunction in men, to increase sexual arousal in women, and asthma.

Panax ginseng is also used for bleeding disorders, loss of appetite, vomiting, intestinal problems, gallstones, bad breath, fibromyalgia, sleeping problems (insomnia), nerve pain, joint pain, dizziness, headache, hearing loss, convulsions, disorders of pregnancy and childbirth, hot flashes due to menopause, common cold and flu, heart failure, high blood pressure, quality of life, wrinkled skin, and to slow the aging process.

Some men apply Panax ginseng to the skin of the penis as part of a multi-ingredient product for treating early orgasm (premature ejaculation).

In manufacturing, Panax ginseng is used to make soaps, cosmetics, and as a flavoring in beverages.

How does it Work?

Panax ginseng contains many active substances. The substances thought to be most important are called ginsenosides or panaxosides. Ginsenosides is the term coined by Asian researchers, and the term panaxosides was chosen by early Russian researchers.

Panax ginseng is often referred to as a general well-being medication, because it affects many different systems of the body.

Uses and Effectiveness?

Possibly effective for:

- Alzheimer's disease: Evidence shows that taking Panax ginseng root daily for 12 weeks can improve mental performance in people with Alzheimer's disease.
- Lung disease called chronic obstructive pulmonary disease (COPD): Taking Panax ginseng by mouth seems to improve lung function and some symptoms of COPD.
- Mental function: Taking Panax ginseng by mouth might improve abstract thinking, mental arithmetic skills, and reaction times in healthy, middle-aged people but not in young adults. Panax ginseng alone does not seem to improve memory. But there is some evidence that a combination of Panax ginseng and ginkgo leaf extract can improve memory in otherwise healthy people between the ages of 38 and 66.
- Erectile dysfunction (ED): Taking Panax ginseng by mouth seems to improve sexual function in men with erectile dysfunction.
- Flu: Taking a specific Panax ginseng by mouth appears to reduce the risk of getting a cold or the flu. But, taking Panax ginseng does not seem to reduce flu symptoms or the length of the illness.
- Multiple sclerosis-related fatigue: Taking Panax ginseng daily for 3 months reduces feelings of tiredness and improves quality of life in females with MS.
- Premature ejaculation: Applying a cream containing Panax ginseng, angelica root, Cistanches deserticola, Zanthoxyl species, torlidis seed, clover flower, asiasari root, cinnamon bark, and toad venom (SS Cream) to the penis one hour before intercourse and washing off immediately before intercourse seems to help prevent premature ejaculation.
- Sexual arousal: Taking powdered Korean red ginseng, a specific form of Panax ginseng, seems to improve sexual arousal and satisfaction in postmenopausal women. Also, using a specific product containing Korean red ginseng and other ingredients (ArginMax for Women, Daily Wellness Company) seems to improve sexual desire in women who report sexual problems.

Ginkgo Biloba

Ginkgo Biloba, or maidenhair, is a tree native to China that has been grown for thousands of years for a variety of uses.

Because it's the only surviving member of an ancient order of plants, it's sometimes referred to as a living fossil.

While its leaves and seeds are often used in traditional Chinese medicine, modern research primarily focuses on ginkgo extract, which is made from the leaves.

Ginkgo supplements are associated with several health claims and uses, most of which focus on brain function and blood circulation.

Here are 12 benefits of ginkgo biloba:

Contains Powerful Antioxidants

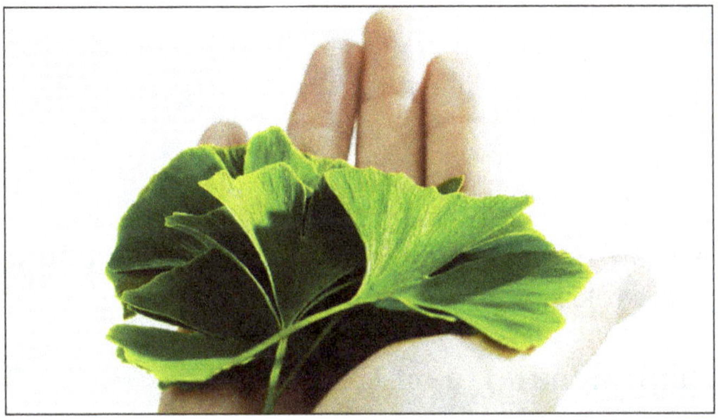

Ginkgo's antioxidant content may be the reason behind many of its health claims.

Ginkgo contains high levels of flavonoids and terpenoids, which are compounds known for their strong antioxidant effects.

Antioxidants combat or neutralize the damaging effects of free radicals.

Free radicals are highly reactive particles that are produced in the body during normal metabolic functions, such as converting food to energy or detoxification.

Yet, they also have the potential to damage healthy tissues, contributing to accelerated aging and disease development.

Research on ginkgo's antioxidant effects is promising. However, it remains unclear exactly how it works and how effective it may be at treating specific diseases.

Can Help Fight Inflammation

Inflammation is part of the body's natural response to injury or invasion by a foreign substance.

In the inflammatory response, various components of the immune system are recruited to fight against the foreign invader or heal the injured area.

Some chronic diseases trigger an inflammatory response even when there is no illness or injury present. Over time, this excessive inflammation can cause permanent damage to the body's tissues and DNA.

Years of animal and test-tube research shows that ginkgo extract can reduce markers of inflammation in both human and animal cells in a variety of disease states.

Some specific conditions in which ginkgo extract has shown to reduce inflammation include:

- Arthritis,
- Irritable bowel disease (IBD),
- Cancer,
- Heart disease,
- Stroke.

While this data is encouraging, human studies are needed before drawing concrete conclusions about ginkgo's role in treating these complex diseases.

Improves Circulation and Heart Health

In traditional Chinese medicine, ginkgo seeds were used to open "channels" of energy to different organ systems, including the kidneys, liver, brain and lungs.

Ginkgo's apparent ability to increase blood flow to various parts of the body may be the origin of many of its supposed benefits.

One study in people with heart disease who supplemented with ginkgo revealed an immediate increase in blood flow to multiple parts of the body. This was attributed to a 12% increase in levels of circulating nitric oxide, a compound responsible for dilating blood vessels.

Similarly, another study showed the same effect in older adults who were treated with ginkgo extract.

Additional research also points to ginkgo's protective effects on heart health, brain health and stroke prevention. There are multiple potential explanations for this, one of which may be the anti-inflammatory compounds present in the plant.

Reduces Symptoms of Psychiatric Disorders and Dementia

Ginkgo has been repeatedly evaluated for its ability to reduce anxiety, stress and other symptoms associated with Alzheimer's disease and cognitive decline associated with aging.

Overall, research results are inconsistent in this area.

Some studies show a marked reduction in the rate of cognitive decline in people with dementia using ginkgo, but others fail to replicate this result.

A review of 21 studies revealed that when used in conjunction with conventional medicine, ginkgo extract may increase functional capabilities in those with mild Alzheimer's.

Another review evaluated four studies and found a significant reduction in a spectrum of symptoms associated with dementia when ginkgo was used for 22–24 weeks.

These positive results could be related to the role that ginkgo may play in improving blood flow to the brain, especially as it relates to vascular types of dementia.

Overall, it's too soon to definitively state or refute ginkgo's role in treating dementia, but recent research is beginning to make this piece clearer.

Improves Brain Function and Well-being

There is some speculation that ginkgo may enhance brain function in healthy individuals.

A handful of small studies support the notion that supplementing with ginkgo may increase mental performance and perceived well-being.

Results from studies like these have given rise to claims linking ginkgo to improved memory, focus and attention span.

However, a large review of research on this relationship concluded that supplementing with ginkgo did not result in any measurable improvements in memory, executive function or attention capacity.

While supplementing with ginkgo may improve mental capability, there are no guarantees.

Can Reduce Anxiety

Some research indicates that supplementing with ginkgo may reduce symptoms of anxiety.

A handful of animal studies have observed reductions in anxiety symptoms that may be attributed to the antioxidant content of ginkgo.

In one study, 170 people with generalized anxiety were treated with either 240 mg or 480 mg of ginkgo or a placebo. The group treated with the highest dose of ginkgo reported a 45% greater reduction in symptoms of anxiety, compared to the placebo group.

While supplementing with ginkgo may reduce anxiety, it's still too early to draw any definitive conclusions from the available research.

Can Treat Depression

A review of animal studies suggests that supplementing with ginkgo may help treat symptoms of depression.

Mice who received ginkgo before an unavoidable stressful situation were less emotionally affected by the stress than the group that did not receive the supplement.

The study indicated that this effect was related to ginkgo's anti-inflammatory properties, which improve the body's ability to cope when stress hormone levels are high.

Nonetheless, depression is a complex condition that may have a variety of root causes.

More research is needed to better understand the relationship between ginkgo and how it may affect depression in humans.

Can Support Vision and Eye Health

Very little research has investigated how ginkgo relates to vision and eye health. However, early results are promising.

One review showed that people with glaucoma who supplemented with ginkgo experienced increased blood flow to the eye, but this didn't necessarily translate to better vision.

Another review of two studies evaluated the effect of ginkgo extract on the progression of age-related macular degeneration. Some participants reported an improvement in vision, but this wasn't statistically significant across the board.

Many of these positive results seem to be related to increased blood flow to the eye.

It's unclear if ginkgo would improve vision in those who don't already suffer from vision impairment.

More research is needed to determine whether ginkgo can increase vision capacity or slow the progression of degenerative eye disease.

Can Treat Headaches and Migraines

In traditional Chinese medicine, ginkgo is a very popular treatment for headaches and migraines.

Very little research is available on ginkgo's ability to treat headaches. However, depending on the root cause of the headache, it may help.

For example, it's well known that ginkgo has anti-inflammatory and antioxidant effects. If a headache or migraine is caused by excessive stress, ginkgo may be useful.

Additionally, if a headache is related to reduced blood flow or constricted blood vessels, ginkgo's ability to dilate blood vessels may improve symptoms.

On the contrary, some migraines are caused by the excessive dilation of blood vessels. In this situation, ginkgo may have little to no effect.

But these examples are just inferences and don't substitute hard evidence.

If you want to try ginkgo for your migraines, it's unlikely that it will cause much harm. Just be aware that it may not necessarily help.

Can Improve Asthma and COPD Symptoms

Some research indicates that ginkgo may improve symptoms of asthma and other inflammatory respiratory diseases like COPD.

This is attributed to the anti-inflammatory compounds in ginkgo, which may allow for reduced inflammation of the airways and increased lung capacity.

One study in 75 people evaluated the use of ginkgo extract alongside glucocorticosteroid medication therapy for managing asthma symptoms.

The levels of inflammatory compounds in the saliva of those who received ginkgo were significantly lower than those who received traditional medication alone.

Another study in 100 people evaluated the use of a mixture of Chinese herbs, which included ginkgo, for treating COPD symptoms.

Those who used the herbal formula reported a considerable reduction in cough and bronchitis at a three-month follow-up, compared to the control group.

At this point, it cannot be determined if this improvement can be attributed to ginkgo alone, or if it was a synergistic effect of the other herbs used in the treatment group formula.

While these results are encouraging, more research on this specific application of ginkgo is needed.

Reduces PMS Symptoms

Preliminary research indicates that ginkgo may help treat both the physical and psychological symptoms of premenstrual syndrome (PMS).

One study in 85 college students revealed a 23% reduction in reported PMS symptoms when consuming ginkgo.

Interestingly, the placebo group in this study also experienced a slight reduction in PMS symptoms, though it was much lower at 8.8%.

Further research is needed to better understand the cause and effect relationship between ginkgo and PMS symptoms.

Treats Sexual Dysfunction

Some sources indicate that ginkgo may treat sexual dysfunction, such as erectile dysfunction or low libido.

Ginkgo has the ability to improve blood levels of nitric oxide, which improves circulation via the dilation of blood vessels.

As a result, ginkgo may also be useful for treating various symptoms of sexual dysfunction by improving blood flow to those areas of the body.

Some research has investigated using ginkgo to treat sexual dysfunction caused by the use of antidepressant drugs (SSRIs). Results indicated that ginkgo wasn't any more effective than a placebo in these cases.

Additionally, there may be an interaction between ginkgo and SSRI medications, which could render them less effective.

One study evaluated the use of ginkgo to increase sexual desire and contentment in women who were concurrently undergoing sexual psychotherapy.

The combination of ginkgo and therapy were effective over a longer term compared to a placebo, but supplementing with ginkgo alone was not.

The rationale for using ginkgo to treat sexual dysfunction makes sense, but research does not support it at this time.

Potential Side Effects

It's important to talk to your doctor before including ginkgo in your routine.

For most adults, the risk associated with taking ginkgo is relatively low, but there are cases in which ginkgo could cause serious harm.

If you are allergic to plants that contain alkylphenols or taking certain medications, you should not take ginkgo.

Possible side effects include:

- Nausea,
- Diarrhea,
- Dizziness,
- Headaches,

- Stomach pain,
- Rash/Allergic reaction.

Ginkgo has the potential to interact unfavorably with certain medications. Some interactions could increase the risk of bleeding.

Possible adverse medication interactions include:

- Blood Thinners (Warfarin, Aspirin),
- SSRIs/MAOIs/Antidepressants (Prozac, Zoloft),
- NSAIDS (Ibuprofen, Tylenol).

Dosage and Supplement Forms

Ginkgo biloba is commercially available in the following forms:

- Capsules,
- Tablets,
- Liquid extracts,
- Dried leaves/Tea.

Most of the current research reflects results used with purified ginkgo extract. Do not eat raw ginkgo seeds, as they are poisonous.

One of the limitations of the studies on ginkgo is that they did not use standardized dosing.

However, the bulk of the evidence seems to support the safety of taking 120–240 mg divided into several doses throughout the day.

There is no clearly defined maximum dosage, but it's wise to start with a lower dose and work your way up to ensure tolerance.

Most research has not evaluated doses greater than 600 mg per day, so it's probably not a good idea to exceed this amount.

Remember, it can take up to six weeks before you begin to notice any effects.

Medicinal Mushrooms

For most species of mushrooms, there is a question as to whether the mushroom is able to treat the diseases/symptoms that have been attributed to it. Unlike microscopic fungi that have yielded some compounds of significance such as penicillin and cephalosporins, many medicinal mushrooms have been utilized as traditional medicine and have never been critically studied to determine if can indeed treat the ailments that have been claimed. Another words, they are comparable to herbal medicine. It is also referred to as Herbalism, Botanical medicine or Herbology and is defined by UK-Skeptics as the use of plants, in a wide variety of forms, for their therapeutic value. Herb plants produce and contain a variety of chemical compounds that act upon the body and are used to prevent or treat disease or promote health and well-being. However, as in the case of medicinal mushrooms, several well known herbals have recently been critically studied, resulting in conflicting conclusions. For example Hypericum perforatum, commonly referred to as St. John's Wort has been used as a herbal since the time of ancient Greece in treatment of depression, but according to the Hypericum Depression Trial Study Group, extracts from this species was ineffective in the treatment of major depressive disorder. However, several European studies have concluded that St. John's Wort was effective in treating mild to moderately severe depression. Why the difference in results and conclusions? Different experimental procedure? poor methodology? For example, China does not use control experimental procedure. Another popular herbal is Ginkgo biloba, which has been demonstrated by Solomon, et al. and Snitz, et al. to not improve memory, attention and enhance cognitive function any more than a placebo. Nevertheless, some species have demonstrated curative properties that have stimulated further studies.

This is similar to what has occurred with medicinal mushrooms. Numerous mushroom species have had various compounds that have been extracted that initially have been demonstrated to have curative properties. However, the initial tests that have been done is based on quick scans for novel compounds that can, for example, inhibit tumors, but these are invivo tests where isolated tumor cells, grown in culture, are tested. While a novel compound may prove effective against the tumor, invivo, that does not mean that it will translate into a useful compound. Think back to antibiotics. When a species was discovered to inhibit/kill bacteria that did not mean that it would become a usable antibiotic for human use. More often than not, the antibiotic was too toxic to even go beyond animal testing. An example of a species that was shown to have initial promise is Calvatia gigantea, during the early years of testing mushrooms for medicinal compounds. Between 1958-1959, Lucas, et al. determined that extracts of this species, named calvacin, contained strong tumor-retarding substances in immature basidiocarps. Roland, et al. continued this line of research by isolating, identifying calvacin and performing invivo test, with cultures of 24 lines of mouse, rat and hamster tumors that demonstrated antitumor activity in 14 of the tumor types. Unfortunately, with the onset of clinical/animal testing, Sternberg, et al. observed numerous side effects, including anorexia, acute liver failure, muscle inflammation and bleeding from the lungs. Some rats receiving the highest dosages administered, died with two days of the experiment.

Mushrooms have been utilized in folk medicine since ancient time. The species of mushrooms used varied in different cultures, i.e. more species have been used in China and Japan than in Western Cultures. It is probable that the difference in usage relates to the mycophilic vs. mycophobic nature of the respective cultures as recognized by Wasson and Wasson. In Western Cultures, the most prominent recognized species and possibly the only one that was identified with any degree of certainty, at the time of the ancient Greeks, was Fomitopsis officinalis. Hippocrates also mentioned fungi and offered their use for certain ailments, but it is unknown as to what species he may have been referring. Dioscorides, a physician around 55 A.D., who is known for his De Materia Medica, the most widely used herbal during his lifetime and for the next 1500 years, had the most influence in Western Culture and probably played a substantial role in the absence of mushroom usage as food as well as in medicine. Pliny and later Galen also held fungi in low esteem. Their opinions, undoubtedly influenced the mycophobic attitude of mushroom in Western Society that continues, to be with us today. However, even they recognized and included F. officinalis among the medicinal plants that they utilized to treat various ailments. Other species utilized for medicinal usage were other bracket fungi; Fomes fomentarius, Phellinus ignarius, Fomintopsis pinicola and others were often used to stop the bleeding and to dress wounds. However, in China, where mushrooms are considered to be the elixir of life, mushrooms have played an important us in medicine for as far back as 7,000 years. Numerous species are recognized, including Lentinula edodes, Hericium erinaceum, Flammulina velutipes, Auricularia polytricha and Tremella fuciformis, to name a few, and these are species that are also prized for eating, as well.

Usage of Medicinal Mushrooms

Most of the benefits that have been attributed to mushrooms and that have been investigated, and studied through the scientific method are those that have been recognized to produce metabolites that inhibit or can destroy cancer cells. Most species that produce these novel compounds do so by what is referred to as immunomodulation, the modification, by suppressing or enhancing immune system and is utilized in treatment of cancerous growth. These compounds include:

Mushroom	Immunomodulating Compound
Lentinula edodes	Lentinan
Schizophyllum commune	Schizophyllan
Grifola frondosa	D-fraction
Coriolus versicolor	PSP (poly-saccharidepeptide) and PSK (also called Krestin)
Ganoderma lucidum	Poly-saccharide (GLPS) fractions

Only a few species containing these compound are being studied. Over 30 species of mushroom have shown anticancer action in animals. PC-SPES, that includes a GLPS fraction, has been demonstrated to control Adenocarcinoma of the prostrate cancer cell line by inhibiting the cell division and growth of their cells. This is a very simple and naive explanation of the mechanism, and there are other various mechanisms by which such compounds have been determined to, but an exhaustive explanation of the various means by which these compounds act is beyond the scope of this course. Various species of mushrooms have been valued as nutritious and tasty food in many parts of the world has been documented by Chang and Hayes in Zaidman, et al. The nutritious property of mushroom is also another means by which they can be benefit the health of the person ingesting mushrooms.

Although there is ample evidence that some mushroom extracts have potentially valuable medicinal properties, none of the compounds are currently approved by the United States Food and Drug Administration (FDA) and still fall under the category of "dietary supplements", as opposed to approved FDA drugs that are prescribed or over-the-counter medication since they have not undergone enough ample testing. This category is also the one that herbals are marketed and must carry the "not approved for use by FDA label". These include such herbals and Echinacea, St. John's Wort, Ginkgo, Fish Oil, Glucosamine, Cordyceps, etc.

Some Examples of Medicinal Mushrooms

Auricularia auricula and A. polytricha: The former species is commonly referred to as Jew's Ear. The common name, according to folklore suggests Judas Iscariot, after his betrayal of Jesus Christ, committed suicide by hanging himself on an elder tree. The ear-like shape of the mushroom is said to be the returned spirit of Judas and serves as a reminder of his betrayal. The species has a temperate distribution as opposed to A. polytricha that has a sub-tropical to tropical distribution. The latter species has a variety of common names, but all have the word "ear" in its name because of the ear-shaped basidiocarp. In Hawai'i, it is referred to as the "pepeiao", the Hawaiian name for ear. Both species belong to the group of Basidiomycota referred to as "jelly fungi" so named because of the consistency of their fruiting body.

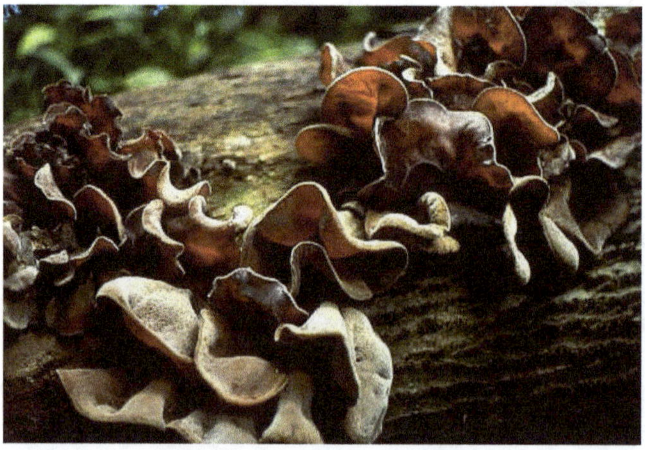

Auricularia polytricha (Pepieau).

Both species have been used in folk medicine in for thousands of years in China and has traditionally been used to treat hemorrhoids and as a stomach tonic. In Europe, A. auricula is boiled in a liquid for inflammation of the throat and for eye irritation. Studies have been carried out that gives evidence that A. auricula may be used to enhance one's immune system. Other studies have demonstrated potential other uses, including the lowering of bad cholesterol, as an anticoagulant and possibly anti-diabetic.

Boletus edulis: This species is commonly referred to as the King Bolete and as the Cepe in Italy. It is a mycorrhizal fungus that is associated with conifers as well as hardwood trees. There are many species of Boletus, but this is probably the most prized species for eating and is also the only species in the genus that has been found to have antitumor properties. In traditional folk medicine, it is also used in treating lumbago, leg pains, numbness in limbs and tendon discomfort to name a few.

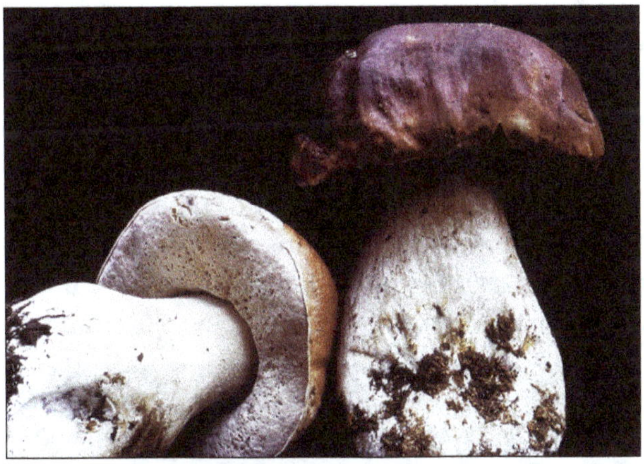

Boletus edulis (Cepe or King Bolete).

Cordyceps sinensis: This species is commonly called the Caterpillar Fungus and has probably been the most extensively studied species. It is a parasitic species that has caterpillar as its host. While it is mostly used medicinally, C. sinensis is also included in some food recipes. It has properties similar to ginseng and is said to be more potent. The first documented of its usage was in 620 AD, during the Tang Dynasty. it has been uses include strengthening of the body after exhaustion or long term illness, impotence, backaches and an antidote for opium poisoning.

A lot of claims made of this fungus. Most of them have yet to be sufficiently investigated. In traditional Chinese medicine, Cordyceps has been used to treat respiratory and pulmonary diseases, e.g. renal, liver and cardiovascular diseases. It is also used in treating immune disorder and has been used in association with cancer chemotherapy treatments and surgery. It is also believed to be a remedy for weakness and fatigue and often used as a "rejuvenator" for increase in energy. Successful treatment for impotence, acting as an aphrodisiac has also been demonstrated in clinical human testing. More can be said, but if even half of the listed treatments are, above, are true, it would indeed be a miracle mushroom.

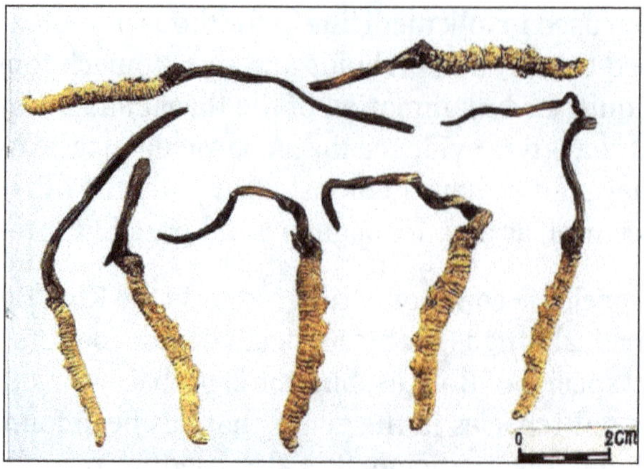

Cordyceps sinensis (Caterpillar Fungus).

Fomitopsis officinalis: A bracket fungus, known under a number of common names, including white agaric, agarick, puring agaric and larch agaric. Aside from its medicinal properties, it has also been used as tinder and also has the common names tinder and touchwood for that reason. This species is probably the oldest traditional medicinal mushroom and was used by both the Greeks and Romans. It was utilized by them as an antidote for poisoning. In later herbals, it was said to be used as a laxative, in preventing flatulence and to rid the intestine of worms and parasites. It was also said to be a successful treatment for malaria, in India. Just prior to the mid 20th. Century, it was still used as a tonic for bronchial asthma and night sweats from tuberculosis.

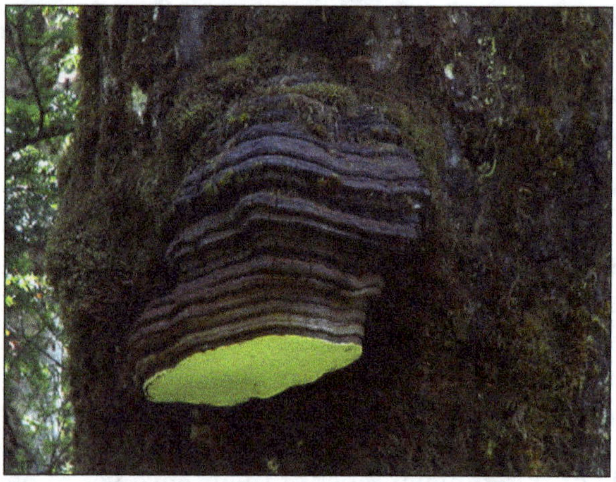

Fomitopsis officinalis (White agaric).

Coriolus versicolor: This is another species of bracket fungus and is commonly referred to as Turkey Tail. It is a common species found world-wide, mostly in temperate regions of the world. The fruiting body has had a number of medicinally useful compounds isolated from it, including the immunoactive PSK and most recently an antitumor polysaccharide that was named coriolan. The PSK has been administered intravenously and orally in human clinical studies of cancer patients and appears to be effective for many forms of cancer, when combined with radiation treatment by enhancing sensitivity of cancer cells to radiation. Survival with treatment of PSK increase survival rate within 5 years was 21% and 52% without.

In traditional Chinese medicine, it is used to reduce phlegm, heal pulmonary disorder, increase energy and benefit people with chronic diseases. In Mexican folk medicine, it has been used to treat ringworm.

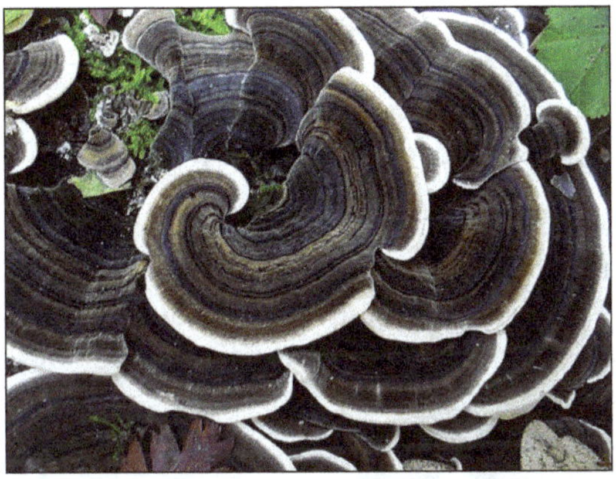

Coriolus versicolor (Turkey Tail).

Lentinula edodes: The shiitake is a mushroom that has been utilized for thousands of years, in Japan and China, for its food value and also prized for its medicinal properties as well. It is also the world's second most cultivated mushroom. In folk medicine, it is said to The shiitake is a well studied medicinal mushroom that has undergone many clinical studies. It has the polysaccharide, lentinan, as well as other polysaccharide that have antitumor properties. Other studies have demonstrated that the shiitake also wards off bacteria that have become resistant to bacteria. For example, patients that had contracted antibiotic resistant strains of Mycobacterium tuberculosis, the causal agent of tuberculosis, had improved their conditions when lentinan was given, and helped limit relapses of tuberculosis in the lungs. Treatment for cancerous liver tumors in rats, liver protection and helped produced antibodies to hepatitis B, lower blood levels of cholesterol and lipids and blood pressure.

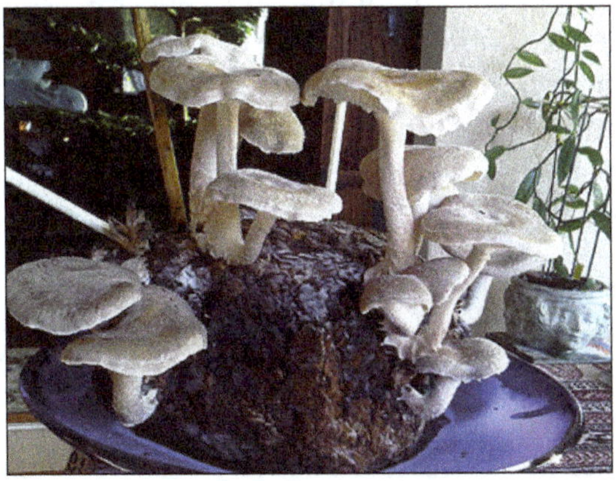

Lentinula edodes (Shiitake).

Tremella fuciformis: This is another species of jelly fungi that is commonly called the snow fungus. This species is found growing on hardwood trees, but is not a wood decomposer as was once thought. Instead, it is a species that is parasitic on hosts that belong the order Xylariales of the phylum Ascomycota. Before the realization of its true nature, cultivation of this species was not possible. It is another of the many Chinese traditional medicinal mushrooms that is said to be able to treat many ailments. These include use as an immune tonic, stops asthma and coughing, reduces phlegem, supports the liver and exhaustion, enhance beauty, reduce fevers, heal ulcers, constipation, abnormal menstrual cycles and many others. This species is found in tropical and temperate areas, throughout the world, on hardwood trees.

In human clinical studies it has been to boost the level of blood cells due to losses from radio- and chemotherapy treatment of cancer patients, boost the immune system by stimulating white blood cell activity. Medicinally, it also been used to lower cholesterol and preventative measures or treatment of cardiovascular problems, such as arteriosclerosis, and abnormal clotting. However, there is no scientific evidence for the latter

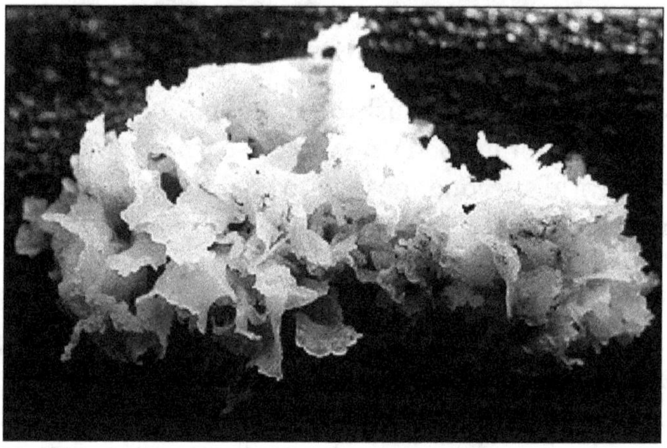

Tremella fuciformis (Snow Fungus).

Ganoderma lucidum: Commonly called the Ling-Zhi in China and Reishi in Japan. This species is one of the bracket fungi, but unlike most species, typically has a long slender stalk that attaches to the side of the "cap" of the fruiting body. This species can be found in North and South America, Europe, Asia on hardwood, especially species of oaks. This species has been utilized in Chinese and Japanese folk medicine for approximately 4000 years, for liver problems, chronic hepatitis, hypertension, arthritis, insomnia, bronchitis, gastric ulcer and asthma.

A number of anti-cancer constituents have been isolated from G. lucidum. These compounds have demonstrated antitumor and immunostimulating activities. Laboratory studies have also shown that this species have anti-allergic activity, bronchitis preventive effect, acts as an anti-inflammatory, antibacterial activities against certain bacteria, lowers blood pressure and has antioxidant activity. Numerous clinical studies have also been carried out and has been shown to be beneficial in treating a variety of disorders.

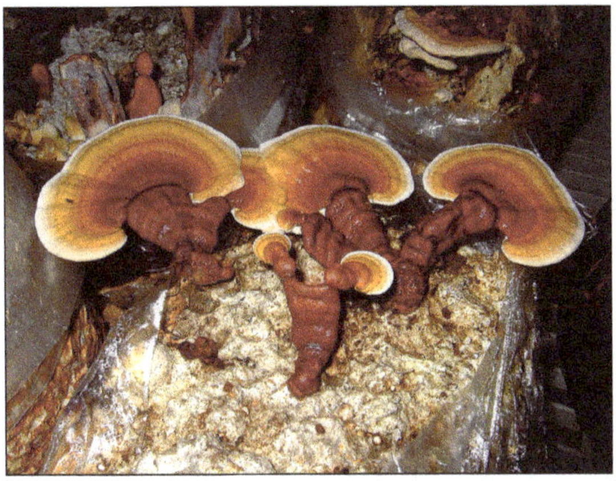

Ganoderma lucidum (Ling-Zhi in China and Reishi, in Japan).

Goji Berries

Goji berries are also known as Lycium barbarum. The goji berry is native to Asia, and people in Asia have been using this brightly colored fruit for more than 2,000 years as a medicinal herb and food supplement. Goji berries are widely available for purchase in health food stores and online.

More recently, supporters have introduced goji berries to the rest of the world with claims of many potential health benefits. Modern science is investigating these claims, and researchers have backed many of them.

Medicinal Benefits of Goji Berries

Here are seven possible benefits of the goji berry with the scientific evidence supporting them:

Protects the Eyes

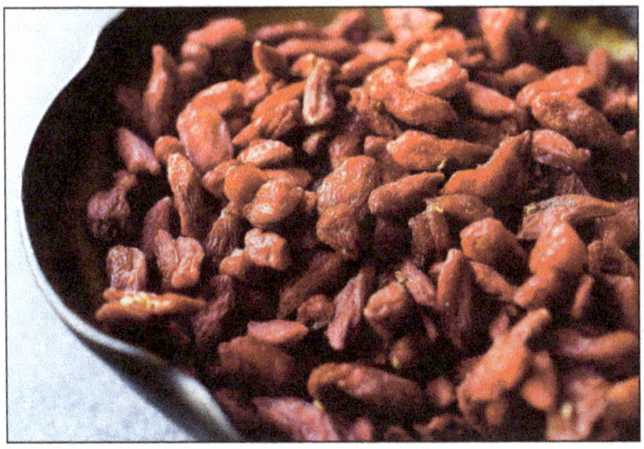

Studies have found that goji berries may help reduce the risk of glaucoma.

Goji berries are believed to protect against age-related eye diseases.

Goji berries can help vision because they contain high levels of healthy antioxidants, especially zeaxanthin.

The same antioxidants can also stop damage from:

- UV light,
- Free radicals,
- Oxidative stress.

One study reported that seniors who drank goji berry juice for 90 days increased zeaxanthin and other antioxidant levels significantly.

A second study shows goji berries protect the retina from the ganglion cells responsible for glaucoma, a condition that can lead to vision loss.

Provides Immune System Support

Goji berries contain healthy antioxidants. Antioxidants are known for their immune-boosting qualities and their ability to fight harmful free radicals and inflammation.

Goji berries contain large amounts of vitamins A and C, similarly to other berries, including blueberries and raspberries. Vitamins A and C are vital for building immunity and preventing illnesses, ranging from the common cold to cancer.

Protects against Cancer

High levels of antioxidants, including vitamin C, zeaxanthin, and carotenoids, are responsible for fighting cancer cells. Antioxidants slow tumor growth, reduce inflammation, and help to remove harmful substances from the body.

Research on mice, finds goji berries may inhibit tumor growth and boost the effectiveness of cancer treatments.

Promotes Healthy Skin

Goji berries contain beta-carotene, which is an essential plant phytochemical. Beta-carotene is known for its ability to promote healthy skin.

Beta-carotene is an ingredient used in skin creams to:

- Improve skin health,
- Reduce skin irritation,

- Manage the effects of the sun,
- Manage the impact of aging.

One study in mice found that when they drank 5 percent goji juice, it gave them enough antioxidants to protect against UV light damage and skin disorders.

Stabilizes Blood Sugar

Goji berries may be helpful in controlling the release of sugar into the blood. Research shows that goji berries balance insulin and glucose levels in the blood.

The same study linked goji berries to increased HDL levels in people with type 2 diabetes. HDL is known as good cholesterol.

Improves Depression, Anxiety and Sleep

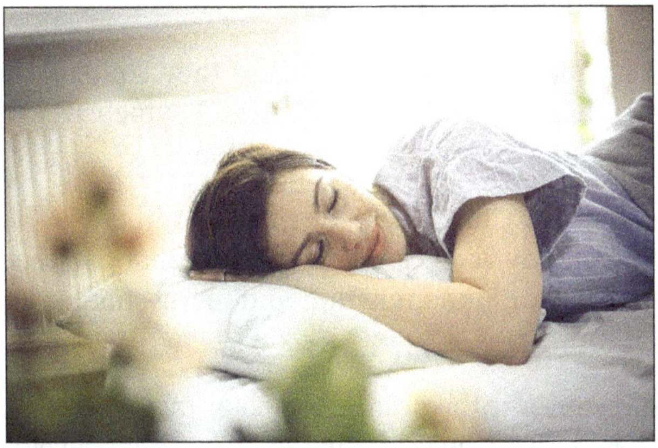

Goji berries may help to improve mood and quality of sleep.

Research that was done using rats shows goji berries can improve depression and anxiety-like behaviors.

Another study in the United States, using humans, also found drinking goji berry juice could improve energy, mood, and digestive health.

In this study, healthy adult participants consumed 120 milliliters of goji berry juice daily or a placebo drink for 14 days.

They completed questionnaires to record their feelings of wellbeing, neurological and psychological health, musculoskeletal symptoms, and digestive and cardiovascular complaints, as well as any adverse effects of the juice each day.

The researchers took measurements to record each participant's blood pressure, body mass, weight, pulse, and vision before and after the 14 days of study.

The group given the goji berry juice reported improved energy, ability to focus, enhanced athletic performance, mental acuity, and feelings of calmness and contentment by day 15.

The study also showed improved quality of sleep in those who consumed the goji berry juice, and none experienced negative effects related to drinking the juice.

Prevents Liver Damage

Goji berries have been used to treat liver disease in traditional Chinese medicine.

Research on animal models indicates goji berries can help with managing liver health and preventing the progression of alcohol-induced fatty liver disease.

Research on human liver cancer cells has also found the goji berry can inhibit tumor growth.

What Makes Goji Berries so Good?

Goji berries are often called a superfood because they contain chemical compounds called phytochemicals that are produced by plants. Phytochemicals in goji berries include polysaccharides, beta-carotene, and zeaxanthin.

Polysaccharides are a primary characteristic of the goji berry. These are an essential source of dietary fiber. A study using aging mice found that polysaccharides in goji berries helped with improving immune function and increasing total antioxidant activity in the body.

Beta-carotene is responsible for the orange-red color pigment in goji berries. Beta-carotene is vital for eye health, bone health, skin health, and cell development. The amount of beta-carotene in goji berries is among the highest of all edible plants.

Zeaxanthin plays a crucial role in supporting the immune system. Many researchers believe that zeaxanthin can prevent macular degeneration, a progressive vision impairment that occurs when the central part of the retina, or macula, deteriorates.

Astragalus

Astragalus is an herb. The root is used to make medicine.

Astragalus is used for many conditions, but so far, there isn't enough scientific evidence to determine whether or not it is effective for any of them.

Astragalus is taken by mouth for hay fever, diabetes, kidney disease, and to strengthen and regulate the immune system.

Some people use astragalus as a general tonic, to protect the liver, and to fight bacteria and viruses. It is also used to prevent and reduce side effects associated with cancer treatment.

Astragalus is commonly used in combination with other herbs.

Astragalus is sometimes applied to the skin to increase blood flow to the area and to speed wound healing.

Astragalus is injected into the vein for the side effects of cancer treatment, heart failure, diabetes, lupus (systemic lupus erythematosus), and many other conditions.

There are several different species of astragalus. Some species contain a nerve toxin and have been linked to livestock poisonings. Some of these species include Astragalus lentiginosus, Astragalus mollissimus, and others. However, these species of astragalus are usually not found in dietary supplements used by humans. Most astragalus supplements contain Astragalus membranaceus.

How does it Work?

Astragalus seems to stimulate and increase the immune system.

Uses and Effectiveness

Possibly effective for:

- Reducing side effects of chemotherapy: Early research suggests that giving astragalus intravenously (by IV) or using Chinese herbal mixtures containing astragalus might reduce nausea, vomiting, diarrhea, and bone marrow suppression (a decrease in the cells that provide immunity) that is associated with chemotherapy treatments.
- Diabetes: Early research suggests that astragalus, given intravenously (by IV) or taken by mouth as a combination product, might help control blood sugar and insulin levels in people with type 2 diabetes.

Atractylodes

Atractylodes is a plant. People use the root to make medicine.

Atractylodes is used for indigestion, stomachache, bloating, fluid retention, diarrhea, loss of appetite, weight loss due to cancer, allergies to dust mites, and joint pain (rheumatism).

Atractylodes is used with other herbs in Traditional Chinese Medicine (TCM) for treating lung cancer (ninjin-yoei-to) and complications of dialysis, a mechanical method for "cleaning the blood" when the kidneys have failed (shenling baizhu san).

How does it Work?

Chemicals in atractylodes might improve function of the digestive tract and reduce pain and swelling (inflammation).

Bupleurum

Bupleurum is a perennial herb that grows mainly in China, but also is cultivated in other areas. The plant grows to approximately 1 m in height and requires abundant sun to flourish. The leaves are long and sickle-shaped with parallel veining. Terminal clusters of small, yellow flowers appear in autumn. The long cone or column-shaped, single or branched root is 10 to 20 cm in length and 0.5 to 1.5 cm in diameter. It is light brown to brown, may be wrinkled, and is easily broken.

Bupleurum is a traditional Chinese herb dating back to the first century BC and is one of the most commonly used herbs in traditional Chinese medicine. One of China's harmony herbs purported to affect organs and energy in the body, bupleurum has been used as a liver tonic, with spleen and stomach toning properties. The plant has also been used to promote perspiration and treat fever, flu, distending pain in the chest, and menstrual disorders.

Coptis Chinensis

Coptis chinensis, also known as the Chinese goldthread, is a species of a flowering plant used in traditional Chinese medicine (TCM). It is, in fact, one of the 50 fundamental herbs of TCM, where it is referred to as huang lian. Widely sold as dietary supplements, extracts, tinctures, and dried whole leaves and roots, Coptis chinensis is often used to treat gastrointestinal disorders and other medical conditions.

Coptis chinensis contains several compounds thought to enhance health, including a salt known as berberine. Berberine belongs to a class of compounds called alkaloids that are known to have antibacterial and anti-inflammatory properties. Berberis has a bright yellow color and is traditionally used as a fabric dye.

Health Benefits

Among TCM practitioners, Coptis chinensis is said to enter the meridians of the heart, large intestines, liver, stomach, gallbladder, and spleen. Because its properties are bitter (astringent) and cold, Coptis chinensis is believed to aid in the treatment of the following conditions:

- Cholera,
- Diabetes,
- Diarrhea ,
- Ear infection,
- Heart disease ,
- High blood pressure,
- High cholesterol,
- Mouth ulcers,
- Respiratory infections,
- Sore throat,
- Vaginal infections.

In addition, Coptis chinensis is believed by some to prevent cancer and protect against liver disease.

There is little evidence that Coptis chinensis offer any health benefits. Most of the research tends to be small or poorly designed with conclusions that are often exaggerated or limited by the size and design of the study.

With that being said, there are some areas of research in which Coptis chinensis offers promise.

Gastrointestinal Health

One of the primary uses of huang lian In TCM is the treatment or prevention of gastrointestinal disorders, including diarrhea, gastroenteritis ("stomach flu"), and bacterial dysentery.

In addition to its antibacterial and anti-inflammatory effects, Coptis chinensis is believed to increase intestinal motility, aiding in digestion and preventing constipation. Sadly, these effects have been little investigated in research.

One key study published reported that rats with chemically-induced sepsis of the gut sustained less intestinal injury if fed Coptis chinensis prior to the induction.

According to the researchers, the rats were fed either a Coptis chinenesis extract containing 9.9% berberine or varying doses of refined berberine. Compared to untreated rats, those treated with supplements experienced little intestine damage due to sharp rises in the antioxidants superoxide dismutase and glutathione peroxidase.

This suggests that Coptis chinensis offers protective benefits to the gut and intestines even in extreme scenarios, such as sepsis.

Diabetes

A number of animal-based studies suggest that Coptis chinensis may have anti-diabetic properties.

According to a 2011 study, rats fed a formulation called Tang-Min-Ling (whose primary ingredient is Coptis chinensis) had less fluctuation in their oral glucose response than rats that were not. This suggests that Coptis chinensis may improve glucose tolerance and aid in the prevention or treatment of type 2 diabetes.

Despite the positive findings, there is no way to know how much Coptic chinensis may have contributed to this effect given that many other herbs (including Chinese skullcap, Chinese rhubarb, and bupleurum) were included in the formulation.

A 2014 review of studies concluded that the evidence supporting the use of Coptic chinensis in treating diabetes "needs to be interpreted with caution." Not only is much of evidence contradictory, but scientists have yet to pinpoint the mechanisms that are said to promote these effects.

Heart Disease

Coptis chinensis may also aid in the treatment or prevention of heart disease, says a 2016 review of studies. It appears to do so, in part, by normalizing blood lipids, including cholesterol and triglycerides.

This, in turn, has a knock-on effect, preventing the buildup of arterial plaque and the development of atherosclerosis while reducing the accumulation of visceral fat.

Berberine is believed to account for many of these effects. In eight of the 43 reviewed studies, berberine appeared to reduce the impact of heart attacks by minimizing collateral tissue damage. With that said, most of the evidence was limited to animal or tissue studies.

Ginger

Ginger is among the healthiest (and most delicious) spices on the planet.

It is loaded with nutrients and bioactive compounds that have powerful benefits for your body and brain.

Here are 11 health benefits of ginger that are supported by scientific research.

Ginger Contains Gingerol, a Substance with Powerful Medicinal Properties

Ginger is a flowering plant that originated from China.

It belongs to the Zingiberaceae family, and is closely related to turmeric, cardomon and galangal.

The rhizome (underground part of the stem) is the part commonly used as a spice. It is often called ginger root, or simply ginger.

Ginger has a very long history of use in various forms of traditional/alternative medicine. It has been used to help digestion, reduce nausea and help fight the flu and common cold, to name a few.

Ginger can be used fresh, dried, powdered, or as an oil or juice, and is sometimes added to processed foods and cosmetics. It is a very common ingredient in recipes.

The unique fragrance and flavor of ginger come from its natural oils, the most important of which is gingerol.

Gingerol is the main bioactive compound in ginger, responsible for much of its medicinal properties. It has powerful anti-inflammatory and antioxidant effects.

Ginger can Treat Many Forms of Nausea, Especially Morning Sickness

Ginger appears to be highly effective against nausea.

For example, it has a long history of use as a sea sickness remedy, and there is some evidence that it may be as effective as prescription medication.

Ginger may also relieve nausea and vomiting after surgery, and in cancer patients undergoing chemotherapy.

But it may be the most effective when it comes to pregnancy-related nausea, such as morning sickness.

According to a review of 12 studies that included a total of 1,278 pregnant women, 1.1-1.5 grams of ginger can significantly reduce symptoms of nausea.

However, ginger had no effect on vomiting episodes in this study.

Although ginger is considered safe, talk to your doctor before taking large amounts if you are pregnant. Some believe that large amounts can raise the risk of miscarriage, but there are currently no studies to support this.

Ginger May Reduce Muscle Pain and Soreness

Ginger has been shown to be effective against exercise-induced muscle pain.

In one study, consuming 2 grams of ginger per day, for 11 days, significantly reduced muscle pain in people performing elbow exercises.

Ginger does not have an immediate impact, but may be effective at reducing the day-to-day progression of muscle pain.

These effects are believed to be mediated by the anti-inflammatory properties.

The Anti-inflammatory Effects can help with Osteoarthritis

Osteoarthritis is a common health problem.

It involves degeneration of the joints in the body, leading to symptoms like joint pain and stiffness.

In a controlled trial of 247 people with osteoarthritis of the knee, those who took ginger extract had less pain and required less pain medication.

Another study found that a combination of ginger, mastic, cinnamon and sesame oil, can reduce pain and stiffness in osteoarthritis patients when applied topically.

Ginger May Drastically Lower Blood Sugars and Improve Heart Disease Risk Factors

This area of research is relatively new, but ginger may have powerful anti-diabetic properties.

In a recent 2015 study of 41 participants with type 2 diabetes, 2 grams of ginger powder per day lowered fasting blood sugar by 12%.

It also dramatically improved HbA1c (a marker for long-term blood sugar levels), leading to a 10% reduction over a period of 12 weeks.

There was also a 28% reduction in the ApoB/ApoA-I ratio, and a 23% reduction in markers for oxidized lipoproteins. These are both major risk factors for heart disease.

However, keep in mind that this was just one small study. The results are incredibly impressive, but they need to be confirmed in larger studies before any recommendations can be made.

Ginger can Help Treat Chronic Indigestion

Chronic indigestion (dyspepsia) is characterized by recurrent pain and discomfort in the upper part of the stomach.

It is believed that delayed emptying of the stomach is a major driver of indigestion.

Interestingly, ginger has been shown to speed up emptying of the stomach in people with this condition.

After eating soup, ginger reduced the time it took for the stomach to empty from 16 to 12 minutes.

In a study of 24 healthy individuals, 1.2 grams of ginger powder before a meal accelerated emptying of the stomach by 50%.

Ginger Powder may Significantly Reduce Menstrual Pain

Menstrual pain (dysmenorrhea) refers to pain felt during a woman's menstrual cycle.

One of the traditional uses of ginger is for pain relief, including menstrual pain.

In one study, 150 women were instructed to take 1 gram of ginger powder per day, for the first 3 days of the menstrual period.

Ginger managed to reduce pain as effectively as the drugs mefenamic acid and ibuprofen.

Ginger may Lower Cholesterol Levels

High levels of LDL lipoproteins (the "bad" cholesterol) are linked to an increased risk of heart disease.

The foods you eat can have a strong influence on LDL levels.

In a 45-day study of 85 individuals with high cholesterol, 3 grams of ginger powder caused significant reductions in most cholesterol markers.

This is supported by a study in hypothyroid rats, where ginger extract lowered LDL cholesterol to a similar extent as the cholesterol-lowering drug atorvastatin.

Both studies also showed reductions in total cholesterol and blood triglycerides.

Ginger Contains a Substance that may Help Prevent Cancer

Cancer is a very serious disease that is characterized by uncontrolled growth of abnormal cells.

Ginger extract has been studied as an alternative treatment for several forms of cancer.

The anti-cancer properties are attributed to 6-gingerol, a substance that is found in large amounts in raw ginger.

In a study of 30 individuals, 2 grams of ginger extract per day significantly reduced pro-inflammatory signalling molecules in the colon.

However, a follow-up study in individuals at a high risk of colon cancer did not confirm these findings.

There is some, albeit limited, evidence that ginger may be effective against pancreatic cancer, breast cancer and ovarian cancer. More research is needed.

Ginger may Improve Brain Function and Protect against Alzheimer's Disease

Oxidative stress and chronic inflammation can accelerate the aging process.

They are believed to be among the key drivers of Alzheimer's disease and age-related cognitive decline.

Some studies in animals suggest that the antioxidants and bioactive compounds in ginger can inhibit inflammatory responses that occur in the brain.

There is also some evidence that ginger can enhance brain function directly. In a study of 60 middle-aged women, ginger extract was shown to improve reaction time and working memory.

There are also numerous studies in animals showing that ginger can protect against age-related decline in brain function.

The Active Ingredient in Ginger can Help Fight Infections

Gingerol, the bioactive substance in fresh ginger, can help lower the risk of infections.

In fact, ginger extract can inhibit the growth of many different types of bacteria.

It is very effective against the oral bacteria linked to inflammatory diseases in the gums, such as gingivitis and periodontitis.

Fresh ginger may also be effective against the RSV virus, a common cause of respiratory infections.

Licorice

Licorice root, also known as sweet root, is used mostly as a sweetener in candies and beverages. People have also used licorice root for centuries for its medicinal benefits.

The medical community is starting to be more accepting of the overall holistic benefits of licorice. However, it's important to note medical research hasn't proved some of these health benefits.

Licorice is available in many forms, either containing glycyrrhizin or as deglycyrrhizinated licorice (DGL).

The word "licorice" refers to the root of a plant called Glycyrrhiza glabra. It's native to Europe and Asia. The plant is actually classified as a weed in those areas.

The early Egyptians loved licorice root. They used it in tea as a cure-all concoction. Licorice was later imported to China where it became an important herb in Chinese medicinal tradition.

Soothes your Stomach

Licorice root is used to soothe gastrointestinal problems. In cases of food poisoning, stomach ulcers, and heartburn, licorice root extract can speed the repair of stomach lining and restore balance. This is due to the anti-inflammatory and immune-boosting properties of glycyrrhizic acid.

One study found that glycyrrhizic acid can suppress the toxic bacteria H. pylori, and can prevent it from growing in the gut. There is also research that's shown people who have peptic ulcer disease, heartburn, or gastritis had improved symptoms when taking DGL.

DGL is the safer form of licorice and can be taken long-term if needed.

Cleanses your Respiratory System

Licorice is recommended to treat respiratory problems. Taking licorice as an oral supplement can help the body produce healthy mucus. Increasing phlegm production may seem counterintuitive to a healthy bronchial system. However, the opposite is true. The production of clean, healthy phlegm keeps the respiratory system functioning without old, sticky mucus clogging it.

Reduces Stress

Over time, stress can leave the adrenal gland exhausted by constantly producing adrenaline and cortisol. Licorice supplements can give the adrenal gland some relief. Licorice root extract can stimulate the adrenal gland, which promotes a healthy level of cortisol in the body.

Assists Cancer Treatment

Some studies say licorice root can potentially aid the treatment of breast and prostate cancers. And some Chinese practices also incorporate it into cancer treatment. The

FDA has yet to approve such treatment methods in the United States. But, research is ongoing, according to the American Cancer Society.

Protects your Skin and Teeth

Topical gels containing licorice are recommended for treating eczema. Licorice can be a successful dermatological treatment due to its antibacterial properties. For that reason, holistic health practitioners often suggest applying licorice to tooth decay to kill bacteria.

Rhubarb

Rhubarb is a plant. The root and underground stem (rhizome) are used to make medicine.

Rhubarb is used primarily for digestive complaints including constipation, diarrhea, heartburn, stomach pain, gastrointestinal (GI) bleeding, and preparation for certain GI diagnostic procedures. Some people use rhubarb so they have to strain less during bowel movements; this reduces pain from hemorrhoids or tears in the skin lining the anal canal (anal fissures).

Rhubarb is sometimes applied to the skin to treat cold sores.

In food, rhubarb stems are eaten in pie and other recipes. Rhubarb is also used as a flavoring agent.

Possibly effective for:

- Stomach bleeding: Taking rhubarb by mouth as a powder or extract seems to help treat stomach bleeding.
- Cold sores: Applying rhubarb along with sage to herpes cold sores seems to improve healing. It might be as effective as acyclovir (Zovirax) cream.
- Kidney failure: Most research suggests that taking rhubarb extract, with or without captopril, improves kidney function in people with kidney failure.

Rehmannia

Rehmannia is a plant. The root and parts that grow above the ground are used to make medicine. Rehmannia is commonly found in herbal combinations used in Traditional Chinese Medicine and Japanese Medicine.

Rehmannia is used for diabetes, "tired blood" (anemia), fever, weakened bones (osteoporosis), and allergies; and as a general tonic.

How does it Work?

There is not enough information to know how rehmannia might work for any medical condition. However, some chemicals in rehmannia seem to affect the immune system and might reduce pain and swelling. Some chemicals in rehmannia also seem to lower blood sugar levels.

Adaptogens

An "adaptogenic" herb helps the human system to adapt, or respond, to demanding and stressful situations. Traditionally, these plants have been used to normalize the function of tissues and organs, helping to increase their efficiency and reduce inflammation. They can often have widely ranging effects, like either raising or lowering blood pressure, depending on the individual. Usually, they are very safe and non-toxic, unlike medicines designed to exploit a specific biochemical mechanism. Many, in fact, are very food-like and probably derived from basic nutritional strategies. Thus, like food, the dose of many adaptogens is relatively high.

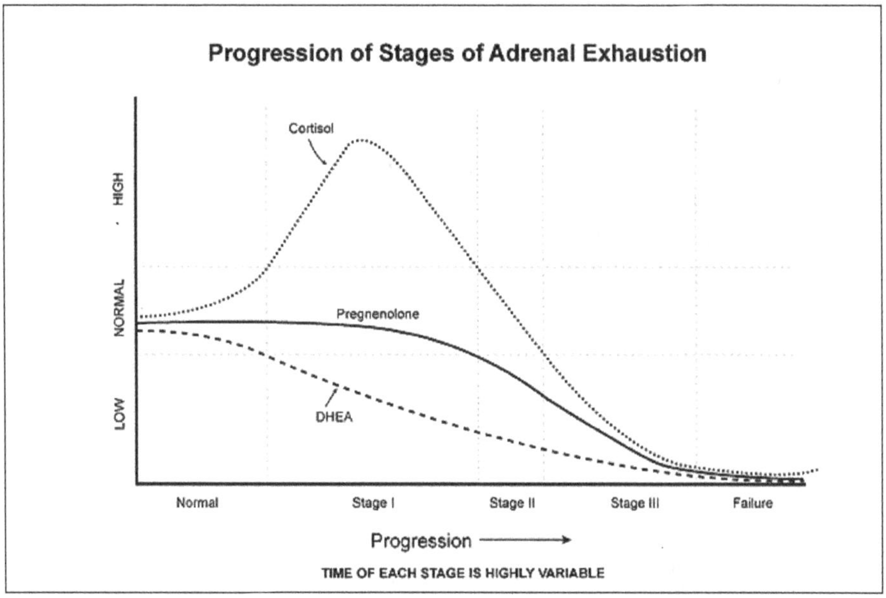

The human physiology responds quite well to external pressure. This response is mediated by the nervous system and adrenal hormones, the most notable being adrenaline and cortisol. Adrenaline's effects are almost instantaneous, and impact all physiological systems, enhancing performance and shutting off digestion. Cortisol's effects peak about 30-40 minutes later, reducing immune-mediated inflammation and raising blood sugar. Repeated stress within 30-60 minutes will see diminished adrenal response, followed by cortisol overproduction; chronic repeated stress will greatly reduce all available hormone levels, leading to exhaustion, depression, anxiety and lack of focus, hormonal disruption, systemic inflammation, insomnia, digestive disturbances, and immune dysfunction.

Adaptogenic herbs can help buffer the stress response, helping to reduce recovery time between stressful events and decrease the system's sensitivity to outside disruption (reducing the perceived frequency of stressful events). Some of their chemistry has been linked to results in vivo (licorice, rhodiola, and the ginsengs for example), but we still know little, from the biochemical perspective, about how they work. So, for best results, it is important to understand a little about herbal and human energetic concepts and the traditional ways of classifying the adaptogenic herbs.

Yang represents activity, movement, high performance, and arousal. It is an energy that is responsible for waking us in the morning, and very much embodied in the adrenal stress response and in fevers. It tends to be warm, dry, and expansive. Yin represents rest, digestion, relaxed awareness, and reduced inflammation. It tends to be cool, moist, and contracting. Both of these energies are required, and they are in constant interplay to maintain a relative state of balance (with occasional excesses of each in turn). These can be seen as two separate adrenal forces, and either one can be excessive, or deficient. The person in question will offer clues as to their energetic balance.

Traditional western herbalism looks at the relative degrees of heat and moisture in an individual, helping with more warming herbs if the person is cool, or moisturizing herbs if there is systemic dryness. Some ideas are listed below. Getting an understanding of the energetic pattern for a person is very useful in selecting the right adaptogen: after all, these plants are classified and known by their energies – that's how they have been studied for thousands of years.

- Yang excess: Red, warm but not dry, loud, active, headaches, night sweats.
- Yang deficiency: Cold, wet and oily, depressed, whispers, fatigue.
- Yin excess: Not cold but very moist, overweight, sluggish, mucus.
- Yin deficiency: Red, neutral to cool, very dry, underweight, panic, insomnia.
- Hot: Red, loud, inflamed (pain, redness), overactive, irritated.
- Cold: Pale, quiet, underactive, stuck, dull pain without redness.
- Dry: Dry skin, irritated eyes, dry cough, constipation, dry mouth.
- Wet: Puffiness (face, hands, tongue, feet), watery discharge, diarrhea.

- Tulsi, Holy Basil (Ocimum sanctum): Delicious as a tea or extract.
- Energy: Cool, well-balanced in moisture, somewhat yin-enhancing.
- Specifics: Inflammation in joints or muscles, autoimmune disease, rheumatism, mood imbalance, gastrointestinal spasm.
- Schizandra (Schizandra chinensis): A powerful berry with a balanced energy profile and incredible taste. Use the extract.
- Energy: Almost perfectly balanced, tends towards moist.
- Specifics: Hormonal disruption, liver disease and dysfunction, skin problems, urinary problems.
- Oats (Avena sativa): Very safe and food-like, the medicinal parts are the unripe seedheads harvested at the 'milky' stage. Use tea or extract, the latter more indicated for acute nervous system symptoms.
- Energy: Moisturizing and somewhat warming, yin-enhancing.
- Specifics: Drained, depleted, dry constitutions, nervous system disruption (depression, anxiety, shock, tremor, pain), menopause.
- Rhodiola (Rhodiola rosea): Enlivening and energizing, provides spark and focus. Use an extract.
- Energy: Neutral to warm, somewhat drying, yang-balancing.
- Specifics: Exhaustion, depression, reduced performance, anxiety, nonspecific pain, lack of focus and poor concentration.
- Korean Ginseng (Panax ginseng): The best Yang tonic. Famous rejuvenator and sexual tonic, used as extract, capsule, or whole root.
- Energy: Warm, yang-enhancing.
- Specifics: Progressive fatigue, sexual deficiency, low libido, depression, digestive disturbances, not for use w/ high blood pressure.

American Ginseng (Panax quinquefolium).

An excellent Yin tonic. Most indicated for today's depleted culture.

- Energy: Neutral, yin-enhancing.
- Specifics: Fatigue, anxiety, insomnia, inflammation, digestive disturbances, immune deficiency with recurrent infection.
- Siberian Ginseng (Eleutherococcus senticosus): Performance-enhancing, for

athletes, students, or those undertaking demanding work. Capsules or extracts are good; a daily decoction is excellent too.

- Energy: Neutral to warm, somewhat yang-enhancing.
- Specifics: Fatigue, repeated stress before total exhaustion, caution w/ high blood pressure.
- Licorice (Glycyrrhiza glabra): Tasty, moisturizing and powerfully anti-inflammatory. Can be taken in any form (as long as it contains the medicinal species).
- Energy: Moist and somewhat cooling, yin-enhancing.
- Specifics: Inflammation and pain, viral co-infection, irritated throat or GI tract, dryness, constipation. Use caution w/ high blood pressure and kidney disease.
- Ashwagandha (Withania somniferum): Ayurvedic "Indian Ginseng". Extract or root powder traditionally mixed with warm milk.
- Energy: Slightly warming, well-balanced, yin-enhancing.
- Specifics: Fatigue with insomnia, weakness and debility after protracted stress or illness.
- Hawthorn (Crategus species):Berry, leaf or flower. The "May Queen" and a premier cardiovascular tonic.
- Energy: Warming, well-balanced.
- Specifics: Cardiovascular disease, depression, lack of focus and anxiety with palpitations, poor circulation.

Medicinal Mushrooms (various species): Mushrooms seem able to balance immune reactions that are complicating the deficiencies and disrupted stress responses that call for adaptogens. Some of my favorites are Red Reishi, especially if there are moist, inflamed allergic symptoms; and Cordyceps, for enhanced stamina and athletic performance.

Decoction

Decoctions are aqueous preparations of plant parts boiled in water for 15–20 min until the water volume is halved. Decoctions are prepared by breaking the plant parts into small pieces before soaking in a given amount of water in an earthenware container (Palayok). The water should cover the plant parts, then the container is covered, and the preparation is boiled until the water volume is halved. The boiled preparation is strained, cooled, and refrigerated which can be kept for 2 or 3 days.

Strong Decoctions

Depending on the type of plant material used, strong decoctions are prepared in two general ways. The first involves boiling the mixture for a longer time. This is usually indicated when working with larger woody pieces of bark. Longer boiling time, up to 2 h or more, is sometimes necessary to break down, soften, and extract the larger pieces. Alternatively, when smaller woody pieces are used yet a stronger remedy is required, the decoction is prepared as above (boiling for 20 min), then it is allowed to sit/soak overnight before straining out the herb. When straining, it is ensured that the cut herb pieces are pressed in the strainer to get as much moisture/decoction out of the herb pieces.

Dried Decoctions

Dried decoctions were developed in Japan in the 1950s and have become a major method of providing herbs in Japan, Taiwan, the United States, and Europe. The dried decoctions are produced by making very large batches of the herb formulas as decoctions (in large tanks), and then draining the liquid from the dregs. The liquid is then evaporated (using heat and vacuum) to form a syrup. The syrup is then put into a spray drier along with a powder carrier (usually starch or the dried, powdered, herb dregs), and the remaining water is evaporated, leaving a dry powder.

Herbal Tonic

Herbal tonics are a potent selection of herbs known to deeply restore, tone, and invigorate multiple body systems. An herbal tonic is a solution or preparation of one or many herbs known to holistically promote health, and be a medicinal source to the mind, body, and spirit.

Many would say that most herbs are tonics. For an herb to be recognized as a tonic, the herb must have been found over many centuries of human use and study to meet specific qualifications. Tonic herbs are said to provide “adaptive energy,” which helps us handle stress much more easily. It is possible to develop a very high degree of adaptability to the many challenges we face and the changes that constantly take place in our lives. By overcoming stressful circumstances successfully, we grow as human beings and we enjoy life much more fully and with radiance. The superior herbs are thus a primary source of true human empowerment. A few keys to knowing about tonic herbs:

- A tonic herb must have anti-aging properties, meaning it is known to support a healthy and long life free of disease.
- A tonic herb must have a profound health-promoting chemistry that produces

noticeable positive health effects within a short period of time after consumption.

- Tonics must help balance physical, emotional, and psychic energy — so as to truly improve one's spiritual well-being and happiness.
- Tonic herbs are known to not have side effects — they are meant to be used over a long time in order for the body to take in long-term benefits. In fact, tonic herbs are known to be gentle and friendly herbs that most, if not all, people can take with no severe effects.
- Most tonic herbs are like foods — they tend to be easily digestible and assimilable; you can add them to your food and drink, enhancing the flavor and effects of any carrier you choose.

Basically, herbal tonics are by definition herbs that safely promote one's health and healthy aging through regular consumption. Tonics are particularly effective because they "teach" the body over time, creating positive effects that eventually operate in the body without the assistance of the tonic. To this day, more and more studies are uncovering the existence of tonic herbs and demonstrating the chemical response they generate in the body over time.

Toxicity and Adverse Health Effects of Some Common Herbal Medicines

In most countries, herbal medicines and related products are introduced into the market without any mandatory safety or toxicological evaluation. Many of these countries also lack effective machinery to regulate manufacturing practices and quality standards. These herbal products are continuously made available to consumers without prescription in most cases and the potential hazards in an inferior product are hardly recognized.

It is important to reiterate the staggering rate at which interest and use of herbal medicines is expanding. Over the past decade, the use of herbal medicines represents approximately 40% of all healthcare services delivered in China while the percentage of the population which has used herbal medicines at least once in Australia, Canada, USA, Belgium, and France is estimated at 48%, 70%, 42%, 38%, and 75%, respectively. In spite of the positive perception of patients on the use of herbal medicines and alleged satisfaction with therapeutic outcomes coupled with their disappointment with conventional allopathic or orthodox medicines in terms of effectiveness and/or safety, the problem of safety of herbal remedies continues to remain a major issue of concern.

The general perception that herbal remedies or drugs are very safe and devoid of adverse effects is not only untrue, but also misleading. Herbs have been shown to be capable of producing a wide range of undesirable or adverse reactions some of which are capable of causing serious injuries, life-threatening conditions, and even death. Numerous and irrefutable cases of poisoning have been reported in the literature.

Aristolochic Acids and Aristolochia Species

Following the discovery of the nephrotoxic and carcinogenic potentials of aristolochic acids, several studies confirmed their genotoxic activity. Schmeiser et al. demonstrated the presence of aristolochic acids-related DNA adducts in renal tissues of patients. These mutagenic adducts when formed are usually poorly repaired and are capable of persisting for years in DNA. Aristolochic acids I and II have been identified in different Asian medicinal plants and also reported to be present in slimming products. This has led to the banning of medicinal products containing these acids in Belgium, UK, Canada, Australia, and Germany.

Misidentification of medicinal plants and mislabeling herbal medicinal products are sometimes responsible for some of the observed adverse events or interaction and that is the reason it is important to assess herbal medicines for possible presence of adulterants. In the UK and many other countries *Aristolochia fangchi* was linked to the development of subacute interstitial fibrosis of the kidney referred to as "Chinese herbs nephropathy". Also, recently a 75-year-old man was reported to have died in Australia from kidney failure associated with a toxic preparation containing the root of *Aristolochia fangchi* which he purchased over the internet for psoriasis. This case report suggested the chronic use of aristolochic acid-containing herbal product as the most likely cause of the patient's death. Similar cases had previously been reported in Taiwan and Japan. Consumption of aristolochic acid-containing Chinese herbal products has also been demonstrated in several studies to be associated with increased risk of urothelial cancer.

A few years back, poisoning that was attributed to Fang-Ji (*Stephania tetrandra* S. Moore) in a weight-loss preparation was actually caused by Guang-Fang-Ji. The presence of aristolochic acids in the latter produced dramatic adverse reactions which led to nephrotoxic and carcinogenic events in more than 100 women using this weight-loss preparation. In this instance, the similarity in the names of the two herbal products was responsible for the confusion and the unfortunate events.

Ephedra Sinica

Ephedra is a very popular herb with long history of traditional use in respiratory conditions. This herb, whose efficacy has been demonstrated in a number of randomized double-blind clinical trials, is currently included in the Chinese Pharmacopoeia for therapeutic use and classified as non-toxic. It is an ingredient in commonly used formulary preparations such as Xiaoqinglong Heji for common cold and Zhisou Dingchuan

Koufuye for asthma. *Ephedra* has been marketed in the US as a weight-loss dietary supplement and its use associated with a number of serious cardiovascular and central nervous systems (CNSs) adverse effects. Several case reports have also linked the use of *Ephedra sinica* and *Ephedra*-containing dietary supplements to adverse events such as hepatotoxicity, neurotoxicity, and transient blindness.

Aconitum Species

Aconitum carmichaeli and Aconitum kusnezoffii are used traditionally for pain relief. The toxicity of the medicinal plants derives primarily from the presence of diester diterpene alkaloids such as aconitine, mesaconitine, and hypaconitine in them. These medicinal plants constitute important ingredients in some commonly used herbal preparations like Sini Tang, Fuzi Lizhong Wan, and Guifu Dihuang Wan for stroke and heart failure, diarrhea and diabetes, respectively. Poisoning due to homemade medicated liquor containing aconite and traditional medicine containing A. carmichaeli were reported in China between 1999 and 2008. Severe cases of cardiac toxicity from consumption of aconitine-containing herbal preparation manifesting as ventricular tachycardia and fibrillation and eventually leading to death have been reported. In other studies bradycardia and hypotension were observed. Clinical cases of aconitine poisoning from A. kusnezoffii consumption have also been reported. Furthermore, the toxic effect of the combination of A. kusnezoffii and A. carmichaeli overdose which manifested as bradycardia and hypotension was also reported by in a case study.

Tussilago Farfara

Traditionally, *Tussilago farfara* has been used effectively for thousands of years for the treatment of acute and chronic cough and it is generally regarded as non-toxic. Total alkaloids and senkirkine isolated from this plant, on the other hand, have been demonstrated to be hepatotoxic. Recently, the potential health effects of the pyrrolizidine alkaloids found in *T. farfara* was reviewed and hepatic veno-occlusive disease and cirrhosis were suggested as the major potential disease outcome in human. However, restrictions in intake of pyrrolizidine-containing herbs and further investigations were recommended because of paucity of data on toxicity assessment in human.

Garlic (Allium Sativum)

Garlic has found relevance for management of hypertension and hypercholesterolemia besides its use as a food or food additive. It is known to contain alliin, which on crushing or chopping in the absence of heat or acid becomes activated by alliinase to allicin. Adverse effects associated with garlic extract including burning sensation in the gastrointestinal tract, nausea, diaphoresis, and lightheadedness have been reported. This extract may also cause contact dermatitis and morbid spontaneous spinal epidural hematoma has been attributed solely to excess garlic ingestion.

Ginkgo Biloba and Ginseng

Ginkgo biloba has found widespread use in a variety of conditions and several products such as elixirs, extracts, tea, as well as capsules and tablets that may differ in terms of content, have been made from the dried root. The whole root which contains ginsenosides is usually used because these compounds possess specific pharmacologic effects that may oppose each other. Over 30 ginsenosides have been identified and these compounds are being investigated for their ability to inhibit cell proliferation, tumor cell invasion, and/or metastasis. Recently, the ability of ginsenosides to modulate signaling pathways involving cell cycle, inflammatory, or growth factor pathways, was demonstrated. The leaf extracts of ginkgo had also been demonstrated to contain active compounds that had found usefulness in improving circulation and cognition.

The plant extracts appear to be relatively safe, although headache, dizziness, restlessness, nausea, vomiting, diarrhea, and dermal sensitivity are the most common side effects that have been observed. Ginkgo has been demonstrated to be capable of inhibiting platelet-activating factor and altering bleeding times. Therefore, cautious use had been advised in individuals or patients on anticoagulants therapy. The ability of ginkgo to induce liver cancer in experimental model was reported recently and genotoxic mechanisms were suggested to play some role in the carcinogenic process. Similar observation was made in the thyroid gland and further studies are required to determine whether the mechanisms for the ginkgo-induced thyroid tumors are also found in humans. In addition to the carcinogenic effects in the liver and thyroid, ginkgo has also been shown to be capable of inducing tumorigenesis in the nasal cavity. The pathogenesis of the nasal lesions was suggested to be related to toxic metabolites of ginkgo reaching the nasal cavity from the systemic circulation. Some other authors, however, have attributed the nasal lesions to gastric reflux/post gavage reflux through the nasopharyngeal duct.

Although, Ginseng products as well as the published descriptions rarely report or specify the species, Ginseng used as herbal remedies has different botanical sources generally obtained from several Panax species including Panax quinquefolius, Panax Ginseng, and Panax pseudoginseng. In large or excessive doses, Ginseng has been reported to cause agitation, insomnia, and elevation of blood pressure while mastalgia and vaginal bleeding have been observed at recommended doses. Other adverse effects that have reported include transient nervousness, excitation, insomnia, inability to concentrate, headache, epistaxis, and allergies. A case of severe but non-fatal Stevens–Johnson syndrome was reported following a 3-day Ginseng administration. Also, spontaneous bleeding from the iris into the anterior chamber of the eye was linked to the use of G. biloba extract.

Kava (Piper Methysticum)

Kava is known for its CNS depressant activity and it is commonly used as an anxiolytic agent. Commonly reported side effects of this medicinal plant include headache, dizziness, gastrointestinal discomfort, and localized numbness after oral ingestion. Large dosages has been shown to be capable of giving rise to dry, scaly skin, and yellowish discoloration of the skin and nails, photosensitivity and redness of the eye. Excessive consumption of kava may also lead to photophobia and diplopia. The muscle relaxant and anticonvulsant effects of this plant have been attributed to its active pyrones constituent. Significant interaction of kava with other CNS depressants which may lead to a comatose state has been reported and as such concurrent use with these agents is usually not advised. In 2002, the US Food and Drug Administration received several reports of liver-related injuries alongside that of a previously healthy young female who eventually required liver transplantation following consumption of kava-containing products. This prompted the FDA to alert consumers on the potential risk of severe liver injury associated with the use of kava-containing dietary supplements. This liver-related risks also prompted regulatory agencies in other countries including Germany, Switzerland, France, Canada, and the UK to warn consumers about the potential risks of kava use and also went on to consider the withdrawal of kava-containing products from the market. In over 25 reports of adverse events outside the US, kava-containing products were associated with liver-related injuries like hepatitis, cirrhosis, and liver failure with some of the affected patients eventually requiring liver transplants.

St. John's Wort

Hypericum perforatum, popularly known as St. John's wort, contains active compounds, such as hypericin, hyperforin, and melatonin. It was once used against viral infections but has gained increased use for mild depressive symptoms. Adverse effects reportedly associated with its use include allergic reactions, headache, dizziness, restlessness, fatigue, dry mouth, nausea, vomiting, constipation, and photosensitivity. Hyperesthesia and a syndrome of dyspnea and hyperventilation with flushing headache, mydriasis, nausea, palpitations, and tremor, have been reported reported a hypomanic episode in a patient with a history of panic disorder who took St. John's wort tincture for 10 days. The hypomanic episode, however, resolved within 2 days of discontinuing the herbal remedy. Interaction of St. John's wort with antidepressants and anticoagulants has been demonstrated and the herbal remedy is usually not recommended in pregnancy because of its uterotonic activity.

References

- Ginkgo-biloba-benefits, nutrition: healthline.com, Retrieved 12 June, 2019
- Atractylodes, vitamins, ingredientmono-1097: webmd.com, Retrieved 09 August, 2019
- The-benefits-of-coptis-chinensis-88938: verywellhealth.com, Retrieved 12 June, 2019
- Licorice-the-sweet-root, health: healthline.com, Retrieved 14 May, 2019
- Rehmannia, vitamins, ingredientmono-1155: webmd.com, Retrieved 27 March, 2019

6

Osteopathy: An Alternative Medicine

Osteopathy is the system of alternative medicine that deals with the treatment of medical disorders by strengthening the musculoskeletal framework. A few aspects that fall under its domain include visceral osteopathy, craniosacral therapy, muscle energy technique, etc. This chapter closely examines these aspects of osteopathy to provide an extensive understanding of the subject.

Osteopathy is a drug-free, non-invasive manual therapy that aims to improve health across all body systems by manipulating and strengthening the musculoskeletal framework.

An osteopathic physician will focus on the joints, muscles, and spine. Treatment aims to positively affect the body's nervous, circulatory, and lymphatic systems.

Manual medicine means that both diagnosis and treatment are carried out with the hands.

Osteopathy is a complementary therapy. It is used alongside conventional treatment to improve health. However, osteopathic physicians are also qualified as medical doctors (MDs), and they have more training than other complementary therapists, such as naturopaths. They specialize in osteopathy.

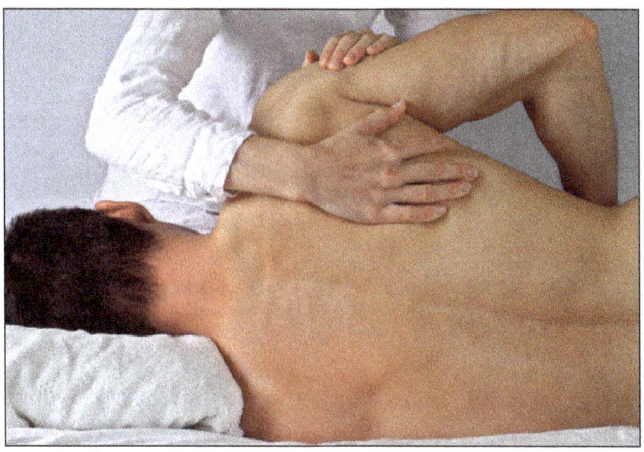

Osteopathy includes manipulation or joints to treat whole systems of the body.

Osteopathy takes a holistic, whole-body approach to healthcare.

It uses manual 'hands-on' techniques to improve circulation and correct altered biomechanics, without the use of drugs.

An osteopathic physician does not concentrate only on the problem area, but uses manual techniques to balance all the body systems, and to provide overall good health and wellbeing.

Diagnosing and treating conditions using these techniques is called Osteopathic Manipulative Medicine (OMM).

Techniques include stretching, gentle pressure, and resistance, known as osteopathic manipulative medicine.

An osteopathic physician may also issue prescription medicine and use surgical methods to support the holistic, manual treatment.

Many osteopathic physicians also serve as primary care physicians in fields such as family medicine, internal medicine, and pediatrics.

Uses

Osteopathy can provide relief and treatment for a wide range of conditions.

These include:

- Arthritis,
- Foot, ankle, hip, and knee pain,
- Back pain, neck pain, and sciatica,
- Hand, shoulder, and elbow pain,
- Headaches,
- Tennis and golfer's elbow,
- Postural problems due to pregnancy, sports injury, driving or work strain, or digestive issues,
- Neuralgia.

Osteopathic physicians can also detect conditions that are not treatable through osteopathy, to refer patients to other specialists.

Physical Examination

The osteopathic physician will physically examine the patient, who may need to remove some clothing to carry out the diagnosis. Patient privacy should be respected during this process.

The examination may take 1 to 2 hours.

The patient will be asked to demonstrate simple stretches and movements to help the osteopathic physician make an accurate analysis of their posture and mobility.

The doctor will also assess the health of the joints, ligaments, and tissues, using a highly trained technique of touch known as palpation.

The osteopathic physician will propose a treatment plan to meet the patient's needs.

This will include the number of sessions likely to be needed, although this number may change depending on the patient's response to treatment.

Osteopathy emphasizes self-healing, so an osteopathic physician may also advise dietary changes, home exercise programs, and lifestyle adjustments.

The manipulation and hands-on work are gentle, but due to the physical work being carried out, a patient of osteopathy may feel sore for the first 24 to 48 hours.

Benefits

Osteopathy can benefit the musculoskeletal framework and other systems.

Osteopathy and Back Pain

Many people approach an osteopathic physician with back pain, but preventive treatment is also possible.

Today's increasingly sedentary lifestyle means that the average American will spend over 10.5 hours per day in front of a screen. This can lead to poor posture and musculoskeletal problems.

Treatment involves gentle and subtle manipulation, especially of the muscles and soft tissues. The doctor may stretch or massage the muscle.

If there are signs of a displaced disk or other serious condition, the osteopathic physician may recommend doing some imaging tests and direct the patient toward conventional treatment.

An osteopathic physician can help prevent problems by pinpointing potential sources of referred pain in good time.

They may suggest dietary modifications and changes to workplace ergonomics, such as seating and desk position.

Prevention advice can involve:

- Stretching exercises,
- Lifting techniques,

- Posture,
- Breathing,
- Stress reduction.

These techniques can help improve posture and reduce pain. Learning to lift with the legs, or example, and to stretch before exercise can reduce injury.

Lifestyle changes can dramatically improve health and reduce ongoing health risks and costs.

Preventing injury means more time keeping active, less time off work, and freedom to enjoy the benefits of healthful living.

Osteopathy and Sleep

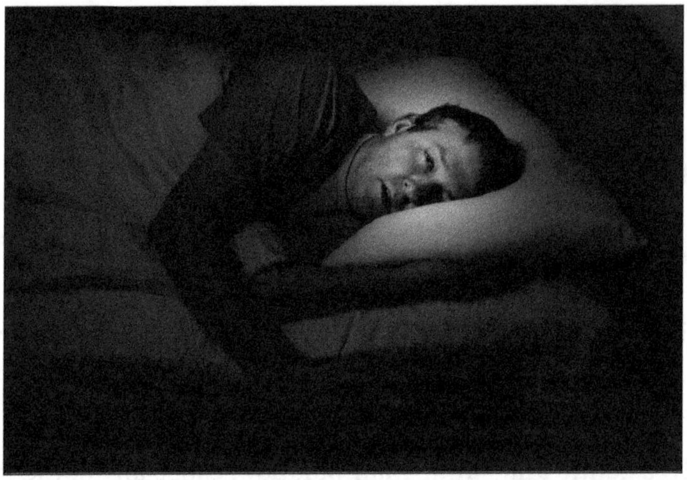

Osteopathy can help a person sleep when chronic pain has been causing insomnia.

Pain and discomfort can lead to a lack of sleep or restless nights.

This can make it harderTrusted Source for the body to function adequately, and reduce the ability to cope with pain.

Osteopathy has been shown to reduce sleeplessness and insomnia resulting from chronic pain.

Studies have shown that osteopathic treatment can reduce sleep apnea in infants under 4 months old.

Other Body Systems

Osteopathic treatments can positively impact the nervous, circulatory, and lymphatic systems, to improve body function and overall health.

Some osteopathic techniques may enhance lymphatic health and bring about internal improvements in the body without needing invasive surgical treatment.

Risks

As with all treatments, osteopathy can involve some risks.

After treatment, it is common for a patient to feel stiff, rather like after exercising, for 24 to 48 hours. Some patients may have a headache for a short while.

Older patients may experience less common side effects, include severe pain, rib fracture in patients with osteoporosis, numbness, and tingling.

If these occur, the patient should speak to their osteopath or their physician.

More severe adverse effects may need emergency medical treatment.

These include stroke, prolapsed disk, pain radiating to a limb, nerve damage, muscle weakness, and bladder or bowel problems.

Visceral Osteopathy

Visceral osteopathy involves a set of therapeutic techniques that correct violation of the functioning of internal organs. Each organ performs a certain movement, dependent or independent of respiration. Disturbances of their natural rhythm lead to functional failures, to occurrence of pain and to development of disease. Movement of organs is structured relative to each other. So failures in one of them inevitably affect the whole system. Before starting treatment, osteopath determines the position of organs and their level of mobility and evaluates the condition of muscle tissue and ligaments. On the basis of the obtained data he diagnoses. The treatment aims at restoring the normal position of organs and bones, strengthening ligaments, improving circulation of lymph, blood and other fluids. As a result of therapeutic effects of the treatment, the body triggers the function of self-healing and development of pathologies stops.

Visceral osteopathy is effective for the following diseases:

- Colitis;
- Ptosis;
- Adhesions;
- Dysfunction of the genitourinary system;
- Gynecological diseases;

- Gastrointestinal problems;
- Disorders in liver and kidneys;
- Insomnia;
- Chronic headaches;
- Varicose veins etc.

The advantage of visceral osteopathy is its complex effect on the body. When working with the internal organs the specialist makes an impact on the spine and bones. Therefore, as a result of treatment the patients get rid of back pain, of spine and often of joints pain.

Visceral osteopathy is effective in the recovery of the body after injury. The techniques are able to correct the displacement of organs, spine and ligaments. Visceral osteopathy treats not only certain diseases, but has a beneficial effect on the organism as a whole. It can help to solve the physiological problems of general nature – to improve the work of joints and bones, nervous system and blood vessels. Visceral osteopathy helps to eliminate many chronic diseases of the abdominal and thoracic cavity. Osteopathic techniques are gentle and easily tolerated by patients of any age.

Craniosacral Therapy

Cranial sacral therapy (CST) is sometimes also referred to as craniosacral therapy. It's a type of bodywork that relieves compression in the bones of the head, sacrum (a triangular bone in the lower back), and spinal column.

CST is noninvasive. It uses gentle pressure on the head, neck, and back to relieve the stress and pain caused by compression. It can, as a result, help to treat a number of conditions.

It's thought that through the gentle manipulation of the bones in the skull, spine, and pelvis, the flow of cerebrospinal fluid in the central nervous system can be normalized. This removes "blockages" from the normal flow, which enhances the body's ability to heal.

Many massage therapists, physical therapists, osteopaths, and chiropractors are able to perform cranial sacral therapy. It can be part of an already-scheduled treatment visit or the sole purpose for your appointment.

Depending on what you're using CST to treat, you may benefit from between 3 and 10 sessions, or you may benefit from maintenance sessions. Your healthcare provider will help you determine what's right for you.

Benefits and Uses

CST is thought to relieve compression in the head, neck, and back. This can soothe pain and release both emotional and physical stress and tension. It's also thought to help restore cranial mobility and ease or release restrictions of the head, neck, and nerves.

Cranial sacral therapy can be used for people of all ages. It may be part of your treatment for conditions like:

- Migraines and headaches,
- Constipation,
- Irritable bowel syndrome (IBS),
- Disturbed sleep cycles and insomnia,
- Scoliosis,
- Sinus infections,
- Neck pain,
- Fibromyalgia,
- Recurrent ear infections or colic in infants,
- TMJ,
- Trauma recovery, including trauma from whiplash,
- Mood disorders like anxiety or depression,
- Difficult pregnancies.

Side Effects and Risks

The most common side effect of cranial sacral therapy with a licensed practitioner is mild discomfort following the treatment. This is often temporary and will fade within 24 hours.

There are certain individuals who shouldn't use CST. These include people who have:

- Severe bleeding disorders.
- A diagnosed aneurysm.
- A history of recent traumatic head injuries, which may include cranial bleeding or skull fractures.

Procedure and Technique

When you arrive for your appointment, your practitioner will ask you about your symptoms and any preexisting conditions that you have.

You'll typically remain fully clothed during the treatment, so wear comfortable clothing to your appointment. Your session will last about an hour, and you'll likely begin by lying down on your back on the massage table. The practitioner may begin at your head, feet, or near the middle of your body.

Using five grams of pressure (which is about the weight of a nickel), the provider will gently hold your feet, head, or sacrum to listen to their subtle rhythms. If they detect it's needed, they may gently press or reposition you to normalize the flow of the cerebrospinal fluids. They may use tissue-release methods while supporting one of your limbs.

During the treatment, some people experience different sensations. These may include:

- Feeling deep relaxation,
- Falling asleep, and later recalling memories or seeing colors,
- Sensing pulsations,
- Having a "pins and needles" (numbing) sensation,
- Having a hot or cold sensation.

Osteopathic Manipulative Medicine Techniques

OMT is a part of the practice of osteopathic medicine that is based on the following four principles: 1) the person is a unit composed of body, mind, and spirit; 2) the body is capable of homeostasis, self-healing, and health maintenance; 3) structure and function are interrelated; and 4) rational treatment is based on an understanding of the above principles. By combining a thorough understanding of anatomy with the pathophysiology of disease, OMT works to restore normal physiological function. The goal of OMT is to treat somatic dysfunction. The *Glossary of Osteopathic Medicine* defines somatic dysfunction as "the impaired or altered function of related components of the somatic system: skeletal, arthroidal, and myofascial structures and their related vascular, lymphatic, and neural elements." Osteopathic physicians use different OMT techniques alone or in combination to resolve somatic dysfunction. Treatments are either "direct," in which the physician engages a patient's restricted plane of motion, or "indirect," in which the body is placed into a position of ease during treatment. OMT requiring a therapeutic correcting force is called an "active" treatment when provided by the physician and "passive" when provided by the patient.

High velocity low amplitude (HVLA): The HVLA technique is a direct, active technique in which the physician engages the pathological barrier of a joint restricted in a normal plane of movement. Once a restricted "barrier" is engaged, the physician employs a quick thrust of short distance through the inhibited plane of motion. The purpose of HVLA is to re-establish normal range of motion by directly engaging the restrictive component of a joint's somatic dysfunction. HVLA is contraindicated especially in patients with cervical rheumatoid arthritis, carotid or vertebrobasilar disease, bony metastasis, and severe osteopenia.

Muscle energy: One cause of somatic dysfunction is postulated to derive from chronically contracted restrictor muscles affecting the body's normal range of movement. Muscle energy is a direct, active treatment with broad applications to any part of the body restricted in motion. In treatment, the physician engages the restrictive barrier and asks the patient to voluntarily move from a precisely controlled position. During the patient's effort, the physician provides an isometric counterforce for 3 to 5 seconds and then allows the muscle to relax for 3 to 5 seconds. A new restrictive barrier is then engaged and the process is repeated 2 to 4 times. Muscle energy increases the length of hypertonic restrictor muscles and allows restoration of normal physiological motion. The mechanism of action of muscle energy is thought to be related to the reciprocal inhibition of agonist/antagonist muscles and the Golgi tendon reflex. When a stretch reflex engages an agonist muscle, its antagonist relaxes via reciprocal inhibition. Similarly, as sufficient tension is placed on the Golgi tendon organ of a muscle, reflex relaxation occurs in the previously hypertonic muscle. Muscle energy is contraindicated in patients with low vitality, fractures, unstable joints, and recent surgery.

Counterstrain: Treatment using counterstrain is directed at discrete areas of tender tissue called tender points. Tender points are painful to the touch and occur in predictable locations throughout the musculature of the body. They are theorized to arise from an antagonist muscle in a state of "panic," lengthening in response to a strained and painful agonist. Counterstrain is an indirect, passive technique in which the patient is positioned away from a restrictive barrier of motion. The physician monitors the tender point in one hand and holds the patient in a position of ease with the other for 90 seconds. By placing the body into a position of maximal ease and comfort, the somatic dysfunction of the strained muscle should begin to resolve. Treatment is repeated until a 70-percent reduction in tenderness is reported by the patient. Tender points can be found in acute and chronic conditions and may be the primary indicator of somatic dysfunction or appear secondary to another medical cause. Absolute contraindications for counterstrain occur in patients with fractures or torn tendons in areas of dysfunction.

Myofascial release: Myofascial release (MFR) is a technique that focuses on fascia and the surrounding muscles. Having found an area of myofascial strain, the physician applies compression or distraction forces to the somatic dysfunction using palpatory feedback to guide the strain to resolution. MFR techniques either directly or indirectly engage restrictive barriers depending on the physician's perceived response of the fascia to palpation. The effectiveness of myofascial techniques is explained via the concept of tensegrity. A tensegrity structure consists of multiple, non-touching rods balanced by a continuous tension system. If one component fails, so does the entire structure. Applying this concept to the human body suggests that bones are the rods and the continuous tension system is the myofascial and ligamentous tissues of the body. Therefore, myofascial strain theoretically has influences across the entire body and resolution allows return of a more balanced homeostatic equilibrium. The use of MFR depends on safe introduction of motion upon dysfunctional tissue. Consequently, MFR is contraindicated for patients with open wounds, fractures, recent surgery, deep vein thromboses, an underlying neoplasm, or other internal injuries.

Craniosacral: Osteopathy in the cranial field was pioneered by a student of A.T. Still's named William Sutherland, DO, and remains one of the more controversial areas of osteopathic manipulative medicine. Central to the cranial technique is the concept of the primary respiratory mechanism, which consists of the inherent rhythmic motion of the brain and spinal cord, fluctuation of cerebrospinal fluid (CSF), mobility of intracranial and intraspinal membranes, the articular mobility of cranial bones, and the involuntary mobility of the sacrum between ilia. The goals of various treatment modalities are to normalize nerve function, eliminate circulatory stasis, normalize CSF fluctuation, release membranous tension, correct cranial articular strains, and modify gross structural patterns. It is important to note that many treatment modalities across the spectrum of OMT are applied to the cranium in addition to those affecting the primary respiratory mechanism. Cranial technique requires special training and should be performed only by certified practitioners. Cranial manipulation is contraindicated for patients with recent trauma, a lack of biomechanical dysfunction or an aversion to receiving treatment.

Lymphatic treatment: Most OMT treatments have an effect on lymphatic circulation. As somatic dysfunction resolves, the body's natural homeostatic mechanisms are normalized and lymphatic drainage is naturally enhanced. However, lymphatic treatments remove impediments to lymphatic flow and augment the clearance of lymph and other immune elements from specific congested tissues. All lymphatic techniques begin with treatment of somatic dysfunction in areas known as "choke points." The three choke points—the thoracic inlet, respiratory diaphragm, and pelvic diaphragm—are areas that can impede lymph between body compartments when dysfunctional. Choke points are treated with MFR assisted by respiration. Once obstruction is reduced, lymphatic treatments employ pumping, soft tissue, and manual drainage techniques to promote fluid movement. Lymphatic techniques are contraindicated in the presence of metastatic cancer, certain infections (e.g., tuberculosis), and hypercoagulable states.

Muscle Energy Technique

Muscle Energy Technique (MET) is a form af a manual therapy which uses a muscle's own energy in the form of gentle isometric contractions to relax the muscles via autogenic or reciprocal inhibition, and lengthen the muscle. As compared to static stretching which is a passive technique in which therapist does all the work, MET is an active technique in which patient is also an active participant. MET is based on the concepts of Autogenic Inhibition and Reciprocal Inhibition. If a sub-maximal contraction of the muscle is followed by stretching of the same muscle it is known as Autogenic Inhibition MET, and if a submaximal contraction of a muscle is followed by stretching of the opposite muscle than this is known as Reciprocal Inhibition MET.

Autogenic and Reciprocal Inhibition

Autogenic and reciprocal inhibition both occur when certain muscles are inhibited from contracting due to the activation of the Golgi tendon organ (GTO) and the muscle spindles. These two musculotendinous proprioceptors located in and around the joints and muscles respond to changes in muscle tension and length, which helps manage muscular control and coordination.

The GTO, located between the muscle belly and its tendon, senses increased tension when the muscle contracts or stretches. When the muscle contracts, the GTO is activated and responds by inhibiting this contraction (reflex inhibition) and contracting the opposing (antagonist) muscle group. This process is known as autogenic inhibition.

The GTO response plays an important role in flexibility. When the GTO inhibits the (agonist) muscle's contraction and allows the antagonist muscle to contract more readily, the muscle can be stretched further and easier. Autogenic inhibition is often seen during static stretching, such as during a low-force, long-duration stretch. After 7 to 10 seconds, muscle tension increases and activates the GTO response, causing the muscle spindle in the stretched muscle to be inhibited temporarily, which makes it possible to stretch the muscle further.

The muscle spindle is located within the muscle belly and stretches along with the muscle itself. When this occurs, the muscle spindle is activated and causes a reflexive contraction in the agonist muscle (known as the stretch reflex) and relaxation in the antagonist muscle. This process is known as reciprocal inhibition.

Types of MET:

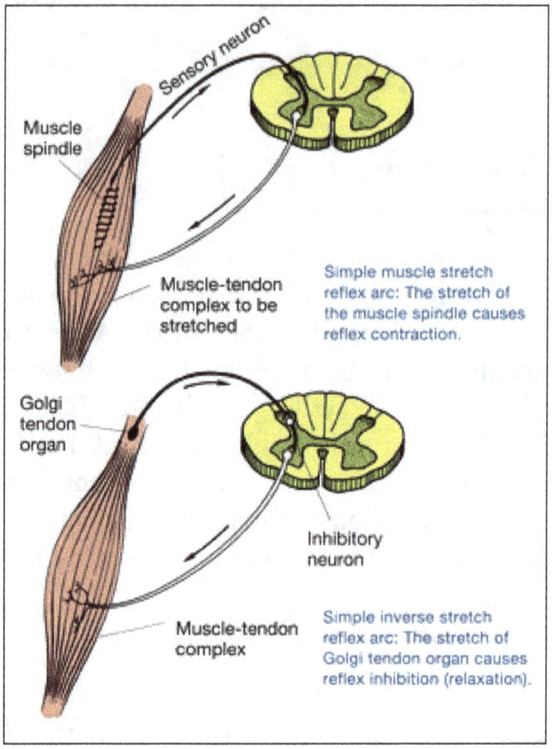

The reflex neuro-muscular inhibition phenomenon.

- Autogenic Inhibition MET.
- Post Isometric Relaxation (PIR) .
- Post Facilitation Stretching (PFS).
- Reciprocal Inhibition MET.

Autogenic Inhibition MET

As already mentioned Autogenic Inhibition METs work on the principle of autogenic inhibition. The two major and well known types of MET that are based on the concept of autogenic inhibition are Post Isometric Relaxation (PIR) and Post facilitation Stretching (PFS).

Post Isometric Relaxation (PIR)

Post Isometric Relaxation is a technique developed by Karel Lewitt. Post Isometric Relaxation (PIR) is the effect of the decrease in muscle tone in a single or group of muscles, after a brief period of submaximalisometric contraction of the same muscle. PIR works on the concept of autogenic inhibition.

The PIR technique is performed as follows:

- The hypertonic muscle is taken to a length just short of pain, or to the point where resistance to movement is first noted.
- A submaximal (10-20%) contraction of the hypertonic muscle is performed away from the barrier for between 5 and 10 seconds and the therapist applies resistance in the opposite direction . The patient should inhale during this effort.
- After the isometric contraction the patient is asked to relax and exhale while doing so. Following this a gentle stretch is applied to take up the slack till the new barrier.
- Starting from this new barrier, the procedure is repeated two or three times.

Post Facilitation Stretch (PFS)

Post Facilitation Stretch (PFS) is a technique developed by Janda. This technique is more aggressive than PIR but is also based on the concept of autogenic inhibition.

The PFS technique is performed as follows:

- The hypertonic and shortened muscle is placed between a fully stretched and a fully relaxed state.
- The patient is asked to contract the agonist using a maximum degree of effort for 5–10 seconds while the therapist resists thepatients force.
- The patient is then asked to relax and release the effort, whereas the therapist applies a rapid stretch to a new barrier and is held for 10 seconds.
- The patient relaxes for approximately 20 seconds and the procedure is repeated between three to five times and five times more.
- Instead of starting from a new barrier, the muscle is placed between a fully stretched and a fully relaxed state before every repetition.

Reciprocal Inhibition MET

Reciprocal Inhibition MET is different from the above two techniques that it involves the contraction of one muscle followed by stretching of the opposite muscle, because contrary to PIR and PFS, Reciprocal Inhibition MET as the name implies is based on the concept of Reciprocal Inhibition.

The Reciprocal Inhibition MET technique is performed as follows:

- The affected muscle is placed in a mid-range position.

- The patient pushes towards the restriction/barrier whereas the therapist completely resists this effort (isometric) or allows a movement towards it (isotonic).
- This is followed by relaxation of the patient along with exhalation, and the therapist applies a passive stretch to the new barrier.
- The procedure is repeated between three to five times and five times more.

Indication

Muscle Energy Techniques can be used for any condition in which the goal is to cause relaxation and lengthening of the muscles and improve range of motion (ROM) in joints. Muscle energy techniques can be applied safely to almost any joint in the body. Many athletes use MET as a preventative measure to guard against future injury of muscles and joints. It is mainly used by individuals who have a limited ROM due to facet joint dysfunction in the neck and back, and for broader areas such as shoulder pain, scoliosis, sciatica, asymmetrical legs, hips or arms, or to treat chronic muscle pain, stiffness or injury.

Permissions

All chapters in this book are published with permission under the Creative Commons Attribution Share Alike License or equivalent. Every chapter published in this book has been scrutinized by our experts. Their significance has been extensively debated. The topics covered herein carry significant information for a comprehensive understanding. They may even be implemented as practical applications or may be referred to as a beginning point for further studies.

We would like to thank the editorial team for lending their expertise to make the book truly unique. They have played a crucial role in the development of this book. Without their invaluable contributions this book wouldn't have been possible. They have made vital efforts to compile up to date information on the varied aspects of this subject to make this book a valuable addition to the collection of many professionals and students.

This book was conceptualized with the vision of imparting up-to-date and integrated information in this field. To ensure the same, a matchless editorial board was set up. Every individual on the board went through rigorous rounds of assessment to prove their worth. After which they invested a large part of their time researching and compiling the most relevant data for our readers.

The editorial board has been involved in producing this book since its inception. They have spent rigorous hours researching and exploring the diverse topics which have resulted in the successful publishing of this book. They have passed on their knowledge of decades through this book. To expedite this challenging task, the publisher supported the team at every step. A small team of assistant editors was also appointed to further simplify the editing procedure and attain best results for the readers.

Apart from the editorial board, the designing team has also invested a significant amount of their time in understanding the subject and creating the most relevant covers. They scrutinized every image to scout for the most suitable representation of the subject and create an appropriate cover for the book.

The publishing team has been an ardent support to the editorial, designing and production team. Their endless efforts to recruit the best for this project, has resulted in the accomplishment of this book. They are a veteran in the field of academics and their pool of knowledge is as vast as their experience in printing. Their expertise and guidance has proved useful at every step. Their uncompromising quality standards have made this book an exceptional effort. Their encouragement from time to time has been an inspiration for everyone.

The publisher and the editorial board hope that this book will prove to be a valuable piece of knowledge for students, practitioners and scholars across the globe.

Index